Vincent Di Stefano has been instrumen
mentary medicine in Australia since the e
of the first peer-reviewed complement;
Journal of the Australian Natural Therapists Ass
member in a number of professional associations representing practitioners
of complementary medicine. He developed and taught programs in pharma-
cognosy and Western herbal medicine at the Southern School of Natural
Therapies and the Australian College of Natural Medicine during the 1980s.
He later served as lecturer in Qualitative Research Methods and History and
Principles of Osteopathy in the Osteopathic Medicine Program at Victoria
University. He was also Course Co-ordinator of the Graduate Diploma of
Western Herbal Medicine and lectured in Philosophical Concepts of
Healing in a number of graduate programs in the Health Sciences
Department at Victoria University. Over the past three decades, he has been
a regular contributor to journals and presenter at conferences and continues
to maintain an active clinical practice in complementary medicine in
Melbourne, Australia.

HOLISM

and

COMPLEMENTARY MEDICINE

Origins and Principles

VINCENT DI STEFANO

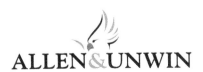

ALLEN&UNWIN

Allen & Unwin
83 Alexander Street
Crows Nest NSW 2065
Australia
Phone: (61 2) 8425 0100
Fax: (61 2) 9906 2218
Email: info@allenandunwin.com
Web: www.allenandunwin.com

National Library of Australia
Cataloguing-in-Publication entry:

Di Stefano, Vincent.
    Holism and complementary medicine : origins and principles.

    Bibliography.
    Includes index.
    ISBN 1 74114 846 4.

    1. Alternative medicine. 2. Alternative medicine - History.
    I. Title.

615.5

Typeset in Centaur MT by Midland Typesetters, Australia
Printed and bound in Australia by Griffin Press

10 9

MIX
Paper from
responsible sources
FSC
www.fsc.org   FSC® C009448

The paper in this book is FSC® certified.
FSC® promotes environmentally responsible,
socially beneficial and economically viable
management of the world's forests.

The caduceus was the magic staff of the Greek god Hermes (Roman Mercury), messenger of the gods. It has been used over the past two centuries as a symbol of healing. This modified image, designed by Linda Robertson, incorporates a plant in place of the second serpent which is traditionally used.

Foreword

Over the last three decades, complementary medicine has been embraced in Western countries across the globe. It is estimated that about 60 per cent of Australians are using complementary medicine, and spend about $A2.3 billion on complementary medicines and the various therapies. In the United Kingdom, it is estimated that about 45 per cent of Britons use complementary medicine, representing some 15 million consultations each year. And in the United States, it has been estimated that $US34 billion is spent annually on complementary medicine.

The rise of complementary medicine in highly developed countries is nothing less than phenomenal. Unlike biomedical health services and pharmaceutical medicines, frequently neither complementary medicine consultations nor remedies receive government subsidy. In spite of this inequity, consumers have been willing to pay for complementary medicines and services out of their own pockets.

Regarded as quacks only a decade ago, complementary medicine practitioners have steadily gained a reputation as primary contact practitioners. The acceptance of complementary medicine in the community is such that complementary medicine courses are now conducted at university level. In spite of this growth, however, scholarly writings on complementary medicine are still limited.

Holism and Complementary Medicine serves to address this deficiency. The author is strategically placed to offer deep insight into complementary medicine practice. He has been involved in complementary medicine education in such areas as naturopathy and herbal medicine since the early 1980s. More recently, he has participated in the design and teaching of undergraduate and graduate programs in Western herbal medicine, philosophical concepts of healing, and qualitative research methods. The perspectives presented in his book have developed from in-depth interviews with a number of highly experienced practitioners and teachers of complementary medicine. They have also been influenced by three decades of community practice in complementary medicine.

This book is divided into two main parts. The first deals with modern complementary medicine practice in a historical context. The second part examines complementary medicine from a medical philosophical perspective. It is often wisely uttered that to understand the present, one must understand the past. The author commences his historical inquiry in Egyptian times, and enthrals the reader with an in-depth comparison between ancient Egyptian medicine practices and today's complementary medicine practice. The reader soon learns that the concept of holism that underpins complementary medicine practice is not a recent development. The author presents solid historical arguments to show that the roots of complementary medicine philosophy are linked to ancient times.

The works of Empedocles, Hippocrates, Theophrastus, Galen and Paracelsus are examined in the light of the development of biomedicine. Contrary to general opinion, biomedicine is not a relatively new phenomenon but rather the legacy of a chain of historical events which evolved essentially around philosophy.

The link between biomedicine, philosophy and science is elaborated upon in much depth. Though biomedicine sees itself resting on the foundations of scientific theory and thought, this text shows how philosophy has greatly influenced and directed the evolution of scientific inquiry over the centuries. It is this same philosophy that has also shaped the development of complementary medicine practice.

The author compares and contrasts the practice of biomedicine and complementary medicine. From one perspective the differences are stark, and this is how many see biomedicine and complementary medicine. But from another perspective, there are surprising parallels. The author draws upon narratives with complementary medicine practitioners and teachers to highlight such issues.

Holism and Complementary Medicine is highly recommended for anyone interested in the historical and philosophical development of complementary medicine. It is a scholarly work that has equal application to undergraduate students, postgraduates, academics, practitioners and consumers of complementary medicine.

Raymond Khoury
Editor, Journal of the Australian Traditional
Medicine Society
July 2005

Contents

Preface

A young man once approached Mahatma Gandhi as he walked alongside a river. The young man bowed respectfully and then began to speak: 'There is so much that needs to be done in this world. There is so much poverty, so much suffering. There is damage to be repaired, there are wrongs to be righted, and there are pains to be healed. How is anyone to be of any help at all?' Gandhi drew the young man's attention to the numerous pebbles that covered the banks of the river and said, 'Find the roundest, the smoothest, the best pebble you can and hold it in your hand. Then select a place in the river that flows before you, take careful aim, and cast the stone towards that spot as accurately as you can. When the pebble hits the water, your work is done. The ripples will do the rest.'

Holism and Complementary Medicine may be likened to a small pebble cast into the stream of a tradition that is as old as the human story itself, the tradition of healing. When confronted with the vast ocean of writings that relate to medicine and healing, and the deluge of articles that regularly wash over readers of the numerous journals devoted to medicine throughout the world, one may well ask, what more is there to be said?

The river never stands still. It runs constantly, flowing around obstacles and receiving the streams that carry water through its endless cycles. Although its composition and shape will often change, its origins remain constant. Every river ultimately draws from the distant headwaters that gather the falling rain. So it is with medicine. Although its forms and methods may change from place to place and from time to time, it draws perennially from the will to alleviate human suffering borne of sickness and disease.

Today, the profession of medicine in the Western world is undergoing a subtle shift in its approach to healing. A widespread reassessment is occurring of the ways in which medicine has been influenced by approaches to health and sickness derived from different methods and world views than those developed by scientific medicine over the course of the past century. This situation stems from a growing realisation that the ways of scientific medicine, though more powerful and impressive than anything that has ever been before, hold their own limitations. This realisation has been significantly hastened by the successes of the modalities of complementary medicine whose approaches to healing often differ significantly from those of Western conventional medicine.

Holism and Complementary Medicine explores the foundational principles underlying many of those approaches. It is hoped that this book will be useful not only to practitioners and students of the healing arts generally, but to all who have an interest in the nature of healing and the principles of physicianship that have guided the mission of medicine throughout history.

This book rests upon the influence and inspiration of those many teachers, colleagues and friends who have, over the past three decades, provided guidance and companionship in the pursuit of the enduring sources of wisdom and healing that have always been part of the story of medicine.

I wish to acknowledge my immense gratitude to a number of friends and colleagues who have generously given of their time and their skill in commenting upon the various chapters of this work. To Peter Ferigno of Victoria University whose wonderfully agile and slippery mind has constantly brought me back to the trees within the forest. To my old friend Paul Hertzog of Monash University who has helped to broaden my understanding of the sincerity and compassion that operates, though often out of sight, within the biomedical project. To my brother in arms, Raymond Khoury of the Australian Traditional Medicine Society, who has provided unswerving support through many projects over the past two decades. His dedication to and perseverance in the causes of herbal and holistic medicine in Australia will be increasingly realised in time to come. To my dharma brother, Paul Orrock of Southern Cross University, whom I have had the great pleasure and privilege of working alongside, and whose clear-minded reflections have helped in the refinement of several chapters. To my former colleague at Victoria University, Bogusha Paks, whose European sensitivities have many times challenged my own assumptions. To Buzz Robertson, who has helped keep me abreast of the times in the ever-changing world of medical literature. To Jenie Stroh of the Southern School of Natural Therapies, who has offered perceptive and constructive reflections on Chapter 5. And to my old friend and sometime mentor, Shuddha Sarma, who early in the piece introduced me to the power and influence of ancient and Eastern systems of medicine and their ways of knowing.

I wish to express my deep thanks to both Annie Gillison and Melanie Guile, who have cast their discerning eyes over the whole manuscript. And also to Rob Campbell whose spirited discussions during our forest walks have helped shape my understanding of the deeper healing towards which we all aspire.

Very special thanks are due to those unnamed respondents who gave so generously of their time and wisdom during the early discussions that brought to light many of the issues raised in Part II of *Holism and Complementary Medicine*. My respondents necessarily remain anonymous for ethical reasons. The italicised quotes used throughout Part II were carefully selected from interview transcripts derived through a qualitative research study undertaken at Victoria University between 1996 and 1998. This study was approved on the understanding that the anonymity of respondents would be respected.

It has been said, 'by teaching I'll be taught'. In confirming the truth of that statement, I remain ever grateful for the energy, the patience and the inspiration of those students who have participated in my various classes during the past twenty-five years of active teaching.

This project may never have come to light were it not for the vision, encouragement and support of the remarkable women of Allen & Unwin. Many thanks to my publisher, Elizabeth Weiss, who has quietly driven the process, to Emma Cant and Emma Sorensen, who tended the refinement of early drafts with patience, to Jeanmarie Morosin, who has orchestrated the production of this book with skill and diligence, and to Jessica Post, who has worked behind the scenes to ensure that the process moved steadily forward.

But my deepest gratitude rests with my loving family, who have weathered my excesses and forgiven my often-extended absences during the making of this text. To my darling Gill, who has ever kept the fires of heart and home burning during this time of exegesis. And to our children Nico, Gina, Luca and Sofia, who have borne my occasional outrages with infinite good grace and humour. My love is ever with you.

VDS

April 2005

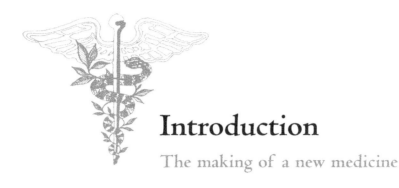

Introduction

The making of a new medicine

Much of the effectiveness of medical people, and much of their acceptance in communities, is a result not of their scientific abilities, but of their commitment to caring, their perceived authority and wisdom, their identification as people privy to arcane knowledge, and perhaps above all, of their willingness to accept (however stressful and unpleasant this might be) responsibility for assuaging grief and offering care even when technological resources are exhausted. These are traditional medical skills, and are at the very heart of the healing project.

G. Allen German, 1987[1]

Suffering is part of the human story. Every one of us has to deal with the reality of birth, sickness and death. Every culture has given rise to those who take on the work of welcoming new life, of helping those who suffer from sickness and disability to regain their health and, at more subtle levels, of giving meaning to the experience of suffering and the limitations that it may bring.

The healing intention has taken many forms throughout history. It has been voiced in the prayers and invocations of countless generations of priests and shamans. It has been carried by the men and women who sought out the substances present in nature and those produced by human ingenuity that help to ease the pain of sickness and hasten the return of health. It continues to find expression in the skill and precision of those dedicated surgeons who daily exercise their art.

Contemporary scientific medicine, also referred to as biomedicine or Western medicine, represents a unique manifestation of the will to heal. It is practised throughout the world, is supported by numerous governments through the funding of educational programs and the provision of resources, and is served by immensely powerful technologies. Practitioners of Western medicine have largely severed ties with their own historic origins. Unlike their Eastern colleagues, Western doctors have by and large put aside both the philosophical understandings and the treatment methods of their forebears.

Both the teaching and the practice of medicine today have become highly standardised throughout the developed world. The curricula of medical programs in universities and medical schools are virtually identical. Every medical graduate emerges from their training with an encyclopedic knowledge of the body and its diseases. The apprenticeships served within urban hospital systems ensure that young doctors are intimately familiar with diagnostic technologies, understand the action and uses of pharmaceutical drugs, and are fully conversant with the surgical procedures commonly used in the treatment of trauma and disease. The practice of medicine in the Western world has, as a consequence, become highly uniform. Any given diagnosis will likely result in a similar prescription or procedure regardless of whether one visits a doctor in Sydney, London, New York or Brussels.

But it is now increasingly understood that scientific medicine represents only one approach to healing, albeit a powerful and unique one. Throughout its brief history, it has been practised alongside other ways of maintaining health and dealing with sickness, even though those ways may have been regarded as marginal and largely irrelevant to the dominant system of scientific medicine.

A surprising cultural development has unfolded in recent decades. Independent practitioners of approaches such as naturopathy, homoeopathy, chiropractic and acupuncture throughout the Western world have attracted the patronage of large numbers of people. Practitioners of scientific medicine were often taken by surprise to learn that their own patients were making use of complementary approaches to healing.

Two decades ago, medical anthropologist Arthur Kleinman laid the cards, as he saw them, on the table:

> The current interest in holistic medicine and alternative healing systems seems best explained as an historically derived populist movement that is perhaps rightly viewed by the medical establishment as anti-professional. Whether this movement is the last bright flicker of a candle about to go out, or represents a major reorientation of how health care will be delivered in our society is a question that the history of the 1980s and 1990s will answer.[2]

In the short time since Kleinman offered his view, that flicker has become a strong flame that now illuminates the path of medicine into the new millennium.

Setting the scene

During the late nineteenth century and the early decades of the twentieth century, medical education underwent a profound transformation. The training of doctors was no longer based upon an apprenticeship system, but became firmly established in science-based programs taught in university environments. Both teachers and students thereby gained access to research facilities and teaching hospitals where patients were available in great numbers.[3] The support of governments in the West was enlisted in this project, based as it was on the foundations of biological science and guided by a highly organised profession of medicine. Earlier traditions of medicine such as herbalism and hygienism, and more recent arrivals such as homoeopathy, Christian Science and chiropractic progressively lost both favour and institutional support. They continued to be quietly practised, however, by a relatively small group of hardy souls who were prepared to weather the isolation of their non-professional and non-aligned status.

Apart from an occasional attack launched by those more vigorous defenders of medical hegemony who periodically came to power in the larger medical associations, a state of relatively benign and peaceful coexistence was reached for much of the first half of the twentieth century. This peace was occasionally tested by some among the ranks of the dispossessed who spoke out too strongly or stridently against the dominant profession. Those who practised outside the mainstream were referred to as quacks at worst, but more often as fringe, unorthodox or lay practitioners.

Things changed dramatically during the 1960s. The formerly inchoate and elusive network of healers and practitioners that had worked unobtrusively within their respective communities began to be identified as 'alternative' healers and were increasingly sought out by more and more people. The term *holistic* was increasingly used to describe such healing approaches. The term itself was not new, but pointed towards an idea that had been first articulated some four decades earlier, and had been slowly configuring ever since.

Holism

Jan Christian Smuts coined the term *holism* in 1925. He used it to describe a philosophical position that was directed towards an understanding of whole systems, rather than particular events or phenomena.[4] Within two years, this new term had made its appearance in the *Encyclopaedia Britannica* and was therein described as 'a viewpoint additional and complementary to that of science'.[5]

Smuts himself was an enigmatic and contradictory character. Born in the British Cape Colony (later to become South Africa) in 1870, he studied law at Cambridge and then returned to his birthplace and a life in politics. He served during the Boer War and proved to be a powerful military strategist, attaining the rank of General. He held office as Prime Minister of South Africa on two separate occasions and was influential in the formation of both the League of Nations and, later, the United Nations. Shortly after the publication of his book *Holism and Evolution* in 1925, he was elected president of the South African Association for the Advancement of Science. In 1930, he accepted the role of president of the Royal College of Science in the United Kingdom.

Smuts repeatedly emphasised that the notion of freedom was integral to any understanding of holism.[6] Yet he held strongly separatist and racist views regarding the rights of blacks in the governance of South Africa, at least during his early years in political office. Smuts also managed to cross swords with Mahatma Gandhi regarding the rights of Indian workers in South Africa.[7]

Although Smuts' early interests revolved around literature, the classics and philosophy, he was drawn strongly to the new vision of reality that began to emerge from the fields of physics and mathematics at the turn of the century. He sought to counter the mechanistic and deterministic view of life that had increasingly dominated the emerging scientific world view by reaffirming the co-centrality of the role of mind and life in creation. For Smuts, the study of matter alone did not provide an adequate understanding of the world. The new physics had opened up a world where matter and energy were interchangeable, and where space and time were no longer separate entities. Through his exploration of 'wholes', Smuts offered a broader and more comprehensive perspective on the nature of reality than that provided by reductionist science.

Smuts' magnum opus, *Holism and Evolution*, came and went largely unnoticed. But the term 'holism' struck a powerful chord that has slowly risen to become a chorus in the intervening decades. Today, holism has come to signify a philosophical position that acknowledges the essential unity of creation. It carries the synergetic understanding that wholes are greater than the sum of their parts.

Holism also recognises that the parts of any given phenomenon may themselves represent whole systems. A molecule of DNA represents a whole system in itself, as does the individual cell that carries the DNA. The organs, made up of numerous individual cells, are each integral systems. And the organism made up of various organ systems is itself a unified whole. Beyond this, the organism itself and the environment within which it is situated are themselves an interconnected unity.

The philosophy of holism can therefore be seen to be complementary to that of reductionism, which holds that phenomena can be understood by an analysis of their individual components. Holism offers a systemic view of reality that acknowledges both autonomy and interdependence, and accepts that matter, life and mind are implicate in and integral to the phenomenal world. It is in this sense that the term holism is used in *Holism and Complementary Medicine*.

Language and labels

Another term that is used consistently throughout this text is *complementary medicine*. Unlike the term *biomedicine*, which keenly identifies the character of contemporary medicine through making explicit its foundational relationship with the biological sciences, the term complementary medicine can be interpreted more as a non-definition, in that it defines itself not by what it is, but by that which it is opposite to, or complements.[8] For the present purposes, complementary medicine will be used as a generic term to describe a number of well-defined approaches to health care whose educational frameworks, underlying philosophies and styles of practice differ from those of biomedicine. Although there are many modalities of healing that may fall within this definition, the term will be used specifically throughout this text to describe the more formalised disciplines of acupuncture and traditional Chinese medicine, naturopathy, homoeopathy, Western herbal medicine and osteopathy, as these represent the particular modalities upon which this inquiry is based.

The term osteopathy as used in this text is to be understood in its common usage in the Australian and British contexts where, unlike in the United States, it refers to both a philosophy and method of treatment derived from the work of Andrew Taylor Still, who developed and promoted it as a comprehensive system of health care during the latter decades of the 1800s.

What was commonly known as alternative medicine during the 1960s and 1970s has since undergone progressive redefinitions on different continents. Much of the discourse relating to non-mainstream medicine during the 1970s and early 1980s centred on the term *alternative medicine*. In the United Kingdom during the 1980s, however, the term complementary medicine gained increasing currency, possibly for political reasons, as 'alternative' may have been perceived as being excessively polarised and as carrying exclusivist undertones in regard to biomedicine. In North America, a peculiar compromise appears to have been settled upon through the use of the term *complementary and alternative medicine* (CAM). The use of the acronym CAM has resulted in a grouping together of what is in actuality a multitude of approaches to health care that differ from biomedicine. Such approaches range from indigenous systems of medicine including Native American medicine, traditional Chinese medicine and Ayurveda, to naturalistic systems such as naturopathy and chiropractic, and may also extend to vibrational medicine, massage and yogic medicine.

More recently, there has arisen from within biomedicine a movement that openly acknowledges the usefulness of many such approaches to healing and health care, and generally supports their incorporation into a broadened base of practice. In Australia and the United States, this development has become known as integrative medicine, while in the United Kingdom it is more commonly referred to as integrated medicine.[9]

In a remarkable social transformation that continues to unfold, what were formerly considered to be marginal and largely inconsequential approaches to health care have unexpectedly gained increasing cultural and legislative endorsement. This transformation has coincided with a noticeable broadening of the philosophical basis of biomedicine, and with a growing acceptance at all levels of other approaches to health care than that of biomedicine.

Changing perceptions

The relationship between biomedicine and its non-mainstream competitors has changed significantly in recent decades. During the 1970s, the rise of what was then referred to as alternative medicine was viewed with suspicion and hostility, and was frequently denounced in the editorials of the learned journals of medicine. During the 1980s, earlier criticisms appeared to gradually soften as an attitude of suspended judgement and cautious appraisal began to develop. During the 1990s, a noticeable shift occurred in the previously rigid boundaries as many within biomedicine took an increasing interest in the possible contribution of such approaches to the health of patients generally.[10]

The disciplines of naturopathy, chiropractic, osteopathy and traditional Chinese medicine have now been formally legitimised in many Western countries by government registration and licensing, and by entry into government-funded university programs. This reality invokes a number of questions. Why has the cultural authority that was painstakingly won by biomedicine over the twentieth century been noticeably eroded? Are there hidden problems within the practice of scientific medicine that the profession itself is blind to? Why do so many choose to make use of the so-called unproven methods of complementary medicine? And at another level, one may ask whether there are common understandings within complementary medicine that differ significantly from those of biomedicine.

Complementary medicine clearly offers something very different from what is provided by scientific medicine. The nature of that difference, however, remains elusive. Certain elements have been tentatively identified in the literature. They include: a differing style of clinical encounter, characterised by longer consultations and a less formal relationship between healer and patient; perspectives on the nature of health and disease that may be more in accord with patients' own views and understandings; an inclination towards health-based rather than disease-based approaches to treatment; a preference for non-pharmacological and non-technological approaches to health care; and an active encouragement and support for patient autonomy.[11]

It has also been suggested that the recent interest in and patronage of practitioners of complementary medicine may simply reflect the exercise of free choice made available by the increased visibility of practitioners of complementary medicine, and a more pragmatic approach to health care based upon patients' experience of benefit from such treatments.[12]

Opening the doors

Holism and Complementary Medicine offers both a journey into the past, and a projection towards the future. But it is essentially grounded in the present time, when the profession of medicine is in the midst of a significant reorientation. This reorientation has been hastened, if not catalysed, by the growing popularity and influence of complementary medicine. This quiet revolution in the way medicine is practised in Western communities is also reflective of an altered world, where many of the certainties of the past have been called into question. The world has changed beyond imagination in recent decades. Many are becoming increasingly aware that the ways of our present civilisation have not necessarily been helpful for the planet or her peoples.

This book does not purport to offer a new or definitive theory regarding the meaning behind the rise of holistic models of healing today. That is a task better left for future commentators who can, with the wisdom of hindsight, interpret more fully the role of complementary medicine in helping broaden the ways in which medicine is both taught and practised in Western communities. What it does offer, however, is an informed exploration of those elements within complementary medicine that have contributed to the movement of large numbers of people in the West towards more holistic approaches to health and healing.

The perspectives presented in *Holism and Complementary Medicine* have been derived from over two decades of personal commitment to the practice and teaching of different aspects of complementary medicine within the Australian context. More importantly, these perspectives have been deepened and refined through collaborative discussions with colleagues who have also served as educator-practitioners of complementary medicine.[13] As such, it offers a unique reflection of those signatory attributes of complementary medicine that differ from those of biomedicine. Those interviewed represent the disciplines of homoeopathy, naturopathy, osteopathy, traditional Chinese medicine and Western herbal medicine. Regardless of the modality practised, every respondent interviewed consistently identified the principle of holism as the underlying philosophical basis of his or her own approach. This principle forms the essential fulcrum around which each of the chapters in Part II turns.

In some ways, this work represents a recovery of lost ground, a re-affirmation of those enduring principles upon which the art and science of medicine have always rested. Those principles include the centrality of the relationship between physician and patient, the dimensions of the task to which the physician is called within that relationship, the philosophical bases of individual systems of healing, and the evolving nature of human conscious-ness and its influence in healing. Each of these elements will be explored in detail in the chapters of Part II. These chapters also offer a detailed overview of the holistic basis of complementary medicine practice, and also deal with those philosophical issues that lie at the heart of any understanding of complementary medicine.

We are, at present, poised at a major turning point in the way that medicine is practised in the Western world. The past century has seen immensely successful developments in new technologies and new methods of treatment. These have made available formerly inconceivable powers of diag-nosis and intervention. Yet despite such prodigious achievements, there are some things that remain constant. Among them is the fact that the practice of medicine is essentially founded on the engagement between two human beings, the physician and the patient, and is not ultimately contingent upon technology or technicianship, although these clearly have had a huge impact on the way medicine is practised today.

The various modalities of complementary medicine are largely out of the loop in regard to their relationship with, or their dependence upon, the powerful technologies of medicine. But they have something very important to offer. They offer both differing perspectives and differing philosophies regarding the nature of life and the nature of health to those held by biomedicine.

Medicine has traditionally drawn as much from philosophy as it has from science. Philosophical issues cannot be put aside as mere abstractions or irrel-evancies in matters of sickness and health. The work of the physician, in all its forms and guises, courts the very limits of our existence. It is implicate in the way we are birthed, the ways in which we deal with the suffering borne of sickness and disease, and the ways that we depart this world.

Our philosophies can help us to connect with each other, with the world in which we find ourselves, and with the many worlds that are available to our belief and imagination. Our lives and experiences cannot be laid open and dissected like cadavers. Although many aspects of life may appear to be predictable, manageable and straightforward, we also live within uncertainty, contradiction, complexity and mystery.

Biomedicine is founded upon an historical pragmatism that has enabled the separation of fact from fancy, of the tangible from the tenuous. Acute care in hospital casualty wards requires immediate and skilled interventions, and not a reflective querying regarding the hidden causes or subtle meanings of a traumatic event. The flow of blood must be staunched. Broken tissues must be tended. Vital signs must be monitored. This is good and necessary. But the art of the healer extends beyond the casualty ward. And it is in such domains that less pressing realities such as the meaning and consequence of sickness episodes, a knowledge of the hidden dimensions of life, and a sensitivity to the subtle influences that condition our health become important. And this is why philosophy is inseparable from medicine.

The three chapters of Part I offer a selective historical review of the progression of the mind of medicine over the past five thousand years of recorded history. The story of healing is, of course, inseparable from the story of humanity, and has been integral to our collective experience since time immemorial. But in the brief review that follows, we are necessarily limited to that which has been transmitted through living traditions and written records.

It has been said that one must know the old in order to understand the new. This will most certainly provide a firm foundation from which to reflect upon the meaning of contemporary medicine. A knowledge of that which has gone before may also provide insight into many of the ideas and philosophies that underlie the various approaches that form part of complementary medicine.

It is important to understand that the ideas and approaches presented in this book do not necessarily reflect the way that complementary medicine is practised on the ground by individual practitioners. Every healer remains free, within reason, to interpret his or her craft in whatever way they choose, once suitably credentialed. This has always been the case. There are many practitioners of complementary medicine who operate in a highly reductionistic manner. Patients are treated according to their presenting symptoms without consideration of cause or consequence. Similarly, there are many holistically inclined practitioners of biomedicine who, while making use of everything scientific medicine can offer, remain acutely sensitive to the more subtle determinants of their patient's health and sickness, and strive to become agents of change in the lives of their patients.

The modernist vision of universal redemption through rationality, scientific thought and technological progress has perhaps been overly optimistic. The growing community support for practitioners of complementary medicine is but one aspect of a widespread cultural response to the problems of modernity. Those problems include a widespread adherence to Cartesian dualism, where matter and mind are seen as separate realms; a masculinism that is reflected in a widespread obsession with control, predictability, and the use of forceful measures to bring about change; the valuation of rationality and intellection over more intuitive and empathic modes of being; and an excessive valuation of materiality over mind and spirit.[14]

This cultural development has led, among other things, to a deepening awareness of the complex of influences that condition our health, and a reconsideration of those sources of healing that are perennially available through simpler means than those offered by technological medicine.

Holism and Complementary Medicine offers a view from the inside of the nature of complementary medicine. It is written in the hope that it may stimulate further studies that explore the experiences of educators, practitioners and patients in the various modalities of complementary medicine. In the longer term, such studies may prove to be far more useful than the myriad clinical and laboratory studies that will doubtless keep researchers busy for decades to come.

~

As many direct quotations from individual respondents inform much of the discussion in Part II, a brief sketch follows of the disciplines taught and practised by those interviewed in order to provide some clarification of their underlying philosophies and treatment approaches. These descriptions are not intended to be exhaustive, but will hopefully be sufficient to provide some insight into the essential character of each approach.

Naturopathy

Naturopathy is a generic term that covers a wide range of modalities including hygienism, nutrition, vitamin and mineral therapy, homoeopathy, herbal medicine, and massage and remedial therapy. Naturopaths therefore represent the general practitioners of natural medicine who are able to utilise a wide range of modalities according to their knowledge and training and the needs of their patients.

Naturopathic philosophy leans strongly towards a vitalist perspective of health and disease. Naturopathic treatment aims to enhance the life force or vitality of the patient through supportive medication and treatment, and through the activation and support of the body's detoxifying capacities. Most practitioners of naturopathy are comfortable with the notion that physical reality is conditioned by an energetic reality that can be utilised for the purposes of healing. The modalities of homoeopathy, acupuncture and vibrational medicine also incorporate such energetic considerations.

Purist metaphors also figure prominently in the naturopathic under-standing of health and disease. The hygienist tradition in particular emphasises this aspect through its encouragement of such practices as periodic fasting and the use of elimination diets. Culturally, however, there are very few who are either prepared to brave such ordeals or to keep a watchful eye on those who would undertake such programs. More commonly, the elimination of toxins is aided through the activation of liver-based detoxification mechanisms and through stimulation of the eliminative capacities of the kidneys, skin and lungs. Attention to such lifestyle issues as diet, physical activity, stress and mental and spiritual orientation are integral to this process.

Naturopathic approaches to health care are essentially educative and transformative in their intent. Patients are actively encouraged to become more informed in such matters as the role of diet and lifestyle upon health and sickness. Philosophically, the naturopathic approach is aligned to an holistic appreciation of our essential connection with nature and natural forces, and seeks through its various methods to enhance our self-healing capacities through the use of natural substances and lifestyle regulation.

Homoeopathy

Homoeopathy was developed in the nineteenth century by the German doctor Samuel Hahnemann. Like Andrew Taylor Still, Hahnemann became deeply disillusioned with the medicine of his day. In his work as a translator of medical texts, he chanced upon the ancient principle of '*similis similibus curentur*', or 'like cures like'. Through a series of early observations on the effects of differing doses of Jesuit bark or *Cinchona officinalis*, prepared according to the peculiar style of homoeopathy, on a group of malaria sufferers, Hahnemann developed a therapeutic epistemology that eventually gave rise to over two thousand homoeopathic remedies. Most of those remedies continue to be used in the homoeopathic materia medica today.

Homoeopathy is essentially a vitalistic system of therapeutics that makes use of medicines prepared through the methods of *succussion* or *trituration*.

The system is based on Hahnemann's observation that minute quantities of substances derived from animal, vegetable and mineral sources, when prepared in a particular way, are capable of curing the pattern of symptoms produced when larger quantities of the same substances are administered.

Homoeopathic medicines are prepared by the serial dilution of plant, animal or mineral products. In real terms, this involves the dilution of one part of starting material with either nine or ninety-nine parts of an inert medium, either a water–alcohol mixture, or sugar of milk powder. This produces what are known as either *decimal* or *centesimal* potencies. The process of succussion, or vigorous shaking, is used to *potentise* liquid mixtures, while the process of trituration, or repeated grinding, is used to potentise solids.

Homoeopaths believe that the strength of action of their medicines increases with each successive dilution despite the fact that there is physically less of the actual starting material. Many of the medicines used by homoeopaths have been so diluted as to contain no trace whatsoever of the original drug or substance used. These higher *potencies* are highly valued by specialist homoeopaths who often speak in glowing terms of their efficacy when used sensitively and appropriately.

Such a notion creates obvious difficulties for any system of medicine grounded in materiality and pharmacology. Not surprisingly, many within biomedicine consider homoeopathy to be a heretical system. This is readily understandable as there are no known conceptual models acceptable to biomedicine whereby the supposed action of homoeopathic remedies can be reconciled with the known laws of pharmacodynamics.

Homoeopaths believe that the potentising process itself releases an energetic template from the starting material. This template is said to be capable of interacting with our own vital energies and thereby exerting a restorative influence on the pattern of symptoms that occur in sickness. Traditional homoeopathic theory also describes a complex system of constitutional tendencies or *miasms* that are said to determine proneness to particular conditions. Again, such a notion finds no resonance in the biomedical paradigm, but is more akin to the qualitative or humoral descriptive systems of Greek, Arabic and Indian medicine.

In actual practice, homoeopathic consultations tend to be lengthy, detailed and very wide ranging. They may explore family history, mental and emotional tendencies, dietary and environmental preferences, and bodily sensitivities in addition to the actual presenting symptoms of the patient. The homoeopathic ideal is to select a specific remedy based upon the patient's symptom picture and constitutional type. When successfully matched, such medicines are said to act in a near-magical way, producing rapid and significant improvement in the patient's condition.

The process whereby homoeopaths arrive at an appropriate remedy is the antithesis of reductionism. That process rests on an exploration of the patient's life-world in such detail as to gain a global view of their physical, mental and emotional attributes. The clinical interaction that characterises the homoeopathic approach is, by its very nature, holistic in character.

Western herbal medicine

Western herbal medicine represents a neglected and devalued repository of much of the knowledge developed over many thousands of years of medical experience in Europe, the Mediterranean and the Americas. Several hundred plant drugs are available to contemporary practitioners of Western herbal medicine as their primary materia medica. Most of these drugs have a long history of traditional use but remain untested according to the current norms of biomedicine. In recent decades, however, increasing interest has been directed towards the nature and activity of a small number of these plant medicines by the medical and scientific community, with the result that their therapeutic usefulness has been validated through clinical trials and their mode of action determined by phytopharmacological investigations.

The philosophical basis of traditional Western herbal medicine is radically different to that of contemporary pharmaceutically based systems of medicine. Like the indigenous systems of Ayurveda and Chinese herbal medicine, traditional European herbal medicine has, for much of its history, leaned heavily upon humoral systems of diagnosis (see Glossary) and treatment derived from the Graeco-Arabic tradition. Plants were thus described in terms of such qualities as heat, cold, dampness or dryness, and prescribed according to interpretations of the patient's symptoms in similar terms. More recently, medicinal plants began to be described according to their perceived actions on the body. Thus they were classified as emetic, soporific, expectorant, demulcent, vulnerary and so on. It is only since the development of the methods of chemistry in the past few centuries that plants have been understood according to the nature of their active chemical constituents.

The practice of Western herbal medicine today can take a number of forms, ranging from a reductionistic pharmaceutical-based approach to more traditional and holistically inclined approaches. The recent investigations that have validated the clinical effectiveness of such plants as *Echinacea* or *Astragalus* as immune system stimulants, *Hypericum* or St John's wort for the treatment of depression, and *Ginkgo biloba* for the treatment of impaired cerebral circulation have led to their promotion and marketing as therapeutic agents for the treatment of specific conditions.

Most contemporary practitioners of Western herbal medicine, however, tend to take a more systemic approach in their work with patients. A patient who presents primarily for treatment of high blood pressure may be prescribed a combination of plant extracts designed to improve the function of the circulatory, nervous and urinary systems. Another suffering from a skin condition may find the focus of treatment directed towards processes of detoxification and elimination through the digestive and urinary systems.

Although most herbalists are aware of the nature of the active constituents in their more powerful plant medicines, carriers of the tradition continue to prescribe plants more on the basis of their actions as nervines, astringents, tonics or demulcents, for example, than upon their chemistry. The treatment itself therefore tends to be directed more towards a restoration of the function of the whole body rather than providing symptomatic treatment for specific conditions.

Most practitioners of Western herbal medicine identify with a holistic philosophy that emphasises the essential unity of human nature and the natural world itself. Plants, as products of nature, are the quintessential medicines of the earth and partake of the same forces that enliven our own nature.

Osteopathy

Osteopathy is a form of structural and functional medicine that was developed in the mid-nineteenth century by the North American doctor Andrew Taylor Still. His confidence in the medicine of the time collapsed after three of his sons died within a short time of each other from meningitis, despite the ministrations of his most trusted and knowledgeable colleagues. Still abandoned his practice of medicine after the death of his sons and spent the next decade immersed in a deep study of human anatomy. He developed a powerful therapeutic system based upon the restoration of structural integrity, and the normalisation of nerve supply, blood supply and lymphatic flow throughout the body.

Traditional osteopathy as described by its originator is both mechanistic and vitalistic. It is mechanistic in the sense that a deep knowledge of anatomical relations informs successful diagnosis and treatment; and vitalistic in the sense that the body is understood to possess inherent healing capacities that are mediated through the circulatory and nervous systems. This capacity for self-healing may, according to osteopathic understanding, be diminished or disturbed by the presence of structural restrictions or *lesions*, and enhanced or restored through structural correction.

In its evolved practice, osteopathy represents far more than a simple mechanistic therapy useful for the treatment of bad backs and sore necks. The body itself is perceived as a holographic *integrum*, and dysfunction in any given part may subtly influence activity in other areas. The purpose of osteopathic examination and diagnosis is to enable the osteopath to identify structural problems that may be influencing joint movement, circulation of the blood, or nerve supply. Through corrective adjustment, the body's self-healing capacity is maximised and enabled to do its work without impediment.

Osteopathic medicine as practised in Australia and the United Kingdom is very different from that currently practised in North America. In Australia and the United Kingdom, osteopathic medicine remains ostensibly a form of manual treatment, whereas in North America osteopathic medicine has in some ways become a more simple, and less technologically oriented, version of biomedicine.

Traditional Chinese medicine

Traditional Chinese medicine represents a well-established cultural system that has been utilised and refined in China over hundreds of generations. Traditional Chinese medicine builds upon a vitalistic and qualitative understanding of human nature and of the influences that sustain life and the phenomenal world itself.

Traditional acupuncture is said to influence the activity of a bipolar energy or *ch'i*, which circulates through a series of channels or *meridians* that interpenetrate our physical bodies. Each meridian is said to be related to a particular organ system or physiological activity. The state of the meridians is assessed by a careful observation of physical signs and by the sensitive reading of the quality of the pulse at a number of positions on the radial artery. The task of the practitioner is to assess the quality and attributes of the energy flowing through the meridians. Any imbalance or disharmony detected is to be corrected by the insertion and manipulation of fine stainless steel needles in selected acupuncture points.

Traditional Chinese medicine also makes use of a vast pharmacopoeia of medicinally active plants that have been used for many centuries. Chinese herbal medicine represents a highly evolved system of internal medicine which is based on a similar understanding to that which informs the practice of acupuncture. Health and disease are diagnosed in energetic terms and plants are selected and prescribed accordingly. This system of medicine has powerful resonances with the Graeco–Arabic medicine that dominated European medicine until the time of the Renaissance. The practice of Ayurvedic medicine, one of the indigenous systems of medicine in India, is similarly based on qualitative principles.

Traditional Chinese medicine rests strongly upon Taoist philosophy which is, by its very nature, holistic. Our human nature participates in the activity and cycles of the natural world. When we live in harmony with nature, we become open systems through which regenerative energies constantly flow. Sickness and disease may reflect disturbances in the free movement of those energies through our bodies. The task of the practitioner is to monitor and interpret the quality of energy flow through the meridian systems, and to correct any imbalance through the use of acupuncture or moxibustion, through the prescription of medicinal substances, through the use of such manual therapies as *tui na*, or through the prescription of such practices as *tai ch'i chuan* or *ch'i gung*.

Although the traditional practice of acupuncture is based on such principles, it can also be applied in a purely symptomatic manner. In the treatment of back pain, for example, the insertion of acupuncture needles into local points without reference to the quality of the pulses or to a general assessment of the quality of energy flow through the meridians often carries significant therapeutic benefits. Similarly, the use of electro-acupuncture for the purposes of surgical anaesthesia represents an independent development that can be interpreted more in neurophysiological than energetic terms.

Traditional Chinese medicine represents an evolved and internally coherent system of therapeutics that has emerged through several millennia of cultural experience. Its methods are based on a different logic to that which underlies Western notions of rationality. Despite this, its inherent efficacy has been acknowledged many times over, and it forms one of the major modalities of complementary medicine that gains increasing Western acceptance even though many aspects of its modus operandi remain uncharted.

PART I
Origins

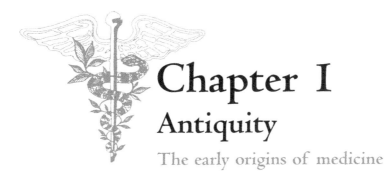

Chapter I
Antiquity
The early origins of medicine

The history of medicine is as much the history of loss of ideas as it is the development of ideas.

David Sobel, 1979[1]

In medicine, we are forever dealing with natural forces, with things in the body we do not understand. But with caution, experience, and discipline, we learn to use these things for the benefit of our patients.

Eric Cassell, 1976[2]

To search out the origins of medicine is to search out the origins of our very humanity. Every culture has its own healing stories. They are carried in the myths that stretch back to times when the world was a fusion of forces and energies that moved us in mysterious ways. Those who could influence those forces became the healers of their respective tribes.

A close study of the principles and practices of any given cultural system of medicine will unearth a commonality that is shared in one way or another with many other systems. The ancient medical texts of India, China and Mesopotamia reveal that the practice of medicine was firmly established many thousands of years ago. Each group had its own herbal pharmacopoeia, its system of dietary regulation, and various restorative practices and rituals. Although each of these cultural groups has given rise to enduring systems of medicine that continue to be practised in modified form even in the present day, the following discussion will focus primarily on those systems of medicine that have specifically influenced the course of Western forms of healing.

We have become accustomed to thinking in very short time frames. Although biomedicine has only been in existence for a little over a century, it is often looked upon as if it has always been around. The medicine of ancient Egypt represents a system that was developed and maintained continuously for a period of more than two thousand years. It served a civilisation that gave rise to extraordinary manifestations of human endeavour in such areas as architecture, navigation, agriculture, metallurgy and social organisation.

As the Egyptian civilisation began to break apart during the time of the Later Kingdoms, many of its medical practices were carried over to Greece. These Egyptian influences, together with elements of Mesopotamian medicine, in turn conditioned the medicine practised in Europe through the Dark and Middle Ages. The medical writings of the Hippocratic school, the texts of Galen and, later, the *Canon* of Avicenna served as primary sources of medical knowledge in European schools of medicine from the time of their establishment during the eleventh century until well into the post-Renaissance period.

The changes that we associate with the development of biomedicine have happened very quickly. They have altered the entire character of the practice of medicine in the developed world. Yet elements of earlier understandings continue to infuse the ongoing practice of medicine in its various modalities both consciously and unconsciously. In the following chapters, we will revisit the movement of Western medicine from the time of the Pharaohs to the present day. That process will enable us to more clearly discern the enduring principles that will always remain relevant to the practice of medicine regardless of our state of technological development or civilisational circumstance.

The medicine of Egypt

Egyptian medicine developed over an immense period of time. Approximately two and a half thousand years passed from the time of the Old Kingdom (approximately 3000 BCE) to the breaking up of the New Kingdom, a few centuries before the birth of Christ.

The magnificent works of architecture that flourished in Egypt were built at great human cost. Many workers were severely injured during the course of their labours. The ancient papyri show us that Egyptian physicians were familiar with both the physical and neurological consequences of bone fractures and other bodily traumas suffered by slaves and construction workers. In their more general healing work, however, Egyptian physicians relied on the availability of many hundreds of medicinal substances. They also called upon the intervention of healing gods whose presence could be awakened through the voicing of spells and the conduct of ritual. The Ebers Papyrus refers to Thoth as physician to the gods. The earth-mother goddess Isis was also venerated for her healing powers; temples of healing built in her name persisted well into the time of the later Kingdoms.

A thousand years before the birth of Christ, Greek physicians in search of knowledge began to make their way to Egypt. Some were to spend time in the temples of Isis. They carried their experiences back to Greece where, within a few centuries, over three hundred temples of healing had been constructed. These were based on similar principles to the healing temples of Egypt, but were dedicated to the Greek god of healing, Asklepias. They were the first hospitals in recorded history.[3]

The ancient texts

Our knowledge of early Egyptian medicine comes from two primary sources. The historical commentaries of Homer, Herodotus, Hippocrates and Pliny offer rich observations of Egyptian culture made over a thousand-year period. More valuable however are the written hieroglyphic records of the Egyptians themselves. Although preserved for thousands of years on the stone walls of pyramids and buildings, and inscribed on numerous papyri and scrolls, the meaning of Egyptian hieroglyphics remained a mystery until the discovery in 1799 of a basalt pillar that was carved as a tribute to Ptolemy V. This pillar, the Rosetta stone, was erected around 200 BCE.

The sides of the pillar were carved in the three scripts that were in common use in Egypt at that time: the hieroglyphs of the Older Kingdoms, the demotic or vulgar later Egyptian glyphs, and the newer Greek characters. Egyptologists carefully compared these three scripts and eventually decoded the carved and painted images that held the stories of ancient Egypt.

Many new papyri were acquired towards the end of the nineteenth century, and archaeologists translated whatever parchments they could find. A few such documents related to the practice of medicine. The most detailed were the two papyri named after their discoverers, Edwin Smith and George Ebers. These are among the oldest written records that tell us how medicine was practised in earlier civilisations. These papyri were destined to open up the complex world inhabited by Egyptian priest-doctors.

The Smith Papyrus, discovered in 1873, was written around 1600 BCE. It carried a great deal of medical knowledge drawn from the records of the Old Kingdom over the previous thousand years. The papyrus consists of a well-preserved roll of parchment 4 metres long, written on both sides. It describes over 700 specific medicines of animal, vegetable and mineral origins that were available to the doctors of the Later Kingdoms. Also included are hundreds of prescriptions, many of which were compounded with rigorous attention to weight and measure of their constituent items.

The huge materia medica of the Egyptian physicians of the New Kingdoms contrasts strongly with the parsimonious repertoire of the Hippocratic physicians of later Greece, who tended to use only a small number of powerful drugs that often contained highly active alkaloids. The final draught of Socrates was prepared from hemlock, or *Conium maculatum*, which contains the deadly alkaloid coniine.

The Smith Papyrus also details a number of surgical cases. These include observations of the effects of head injuries such as skull fractures and sword strokes to the face and scalp, and describe fractures of long bones. Egyptian doctors recognised early that dislocations and fractures of the bones of the neck often resulted in paralysis or partial paralysis of the arms, legs and body sphincters. They also observed that such injuries usually had a poor prognosis. These observations were made during the time of the Old Kingdom, between 3000 and 2400 BCE, and were incorporated early into the texts of medicine used in the later teaching academies.

The reverse side of the Smith Papyrus describes the very different style of medicine that developed in subsequent centuries. This section was written sometime between 1600 and 1200 BCE. It details numerous substances used as medicines, and records many of the invocations, spells and hymns that were used in times of plague and sickness.

In 1872, a year before Edwin Smith found this priceless document, the Egyptologist George Ebers chanced upon another major papyrus while on his travels. On later translation, this proved to be an encyclopaedic compilation of medical knowledge from the Old and Middle Kingdom periods. It was written around 1600 BCE and is four times the length of the Smith Papyrus. It is believed to have been an important instructional text in the *Pir Ankh*, the 'Houses of Life' or sacred academies of learning. The Ebers Papyrus, as it became known, begins with a series of invocations and spells, and then goes on to describe many hundreds of formulae for medicines. It also details symptom pictures and treatment methods for a range of named conditions.

These two papyri and a small number of other preserved medical texts from ancient Egypt have provided us with considerable knowledge of the lived world of Egyptian doctors and their patients.

Priest and doctor

Early Egyptian medicine was ruled by a priestly caste. Disease was viewed as a bodily invasion by demonic influences that could create disturbance and disease. The task of the priest-doctor was to drive out such influences.

Doctors were trained to use their voices in the invocation of healing forces. Diagnosis largely consisted in the naming of the disease or of the demonic presence responsible for the disease. Treatment methods involved both the use of drugs and the commanding of the offending disease or spirit to depart from the patient. Such commands were probably accompanied by the ritual movement and dramatic vocalisations that are often a part of shamanic approaches to healing.

Those poor unfortunates deemed to be insane or possessed by evil spirits were dealt the worst of medicines. The most bitter and unpalatable plants available were often compounded with animal urine or faeces. Such 'medicines' were considered sufficiently shocking to drive out even the worst of demons. In more recent times, Western psychiatrists devised similarly extreme interventions, such as shock treatment (ECT) and surgical excision of the frontal cortex of the brain (pre-frontal lobotomy) to deal with intractable mental afflictions.

The Ebers Papyrus describes the preparation and use of many vegetable and mineral medicines. These include agents prepared from colchicum, gentian, castor oil and opium. The ores of antimony, lead and copper were also used in the preparation of medicines. And as noted earlier, doctors at the time were not averse to using such choice items as the blood, excreta, fats and viscera of birds, mammals and reptiles.

Despite the post-mortem manipulations of mummification, only a vague and rudimentary knowledge of anatomy was ever developed by the Egyptians. Although there were general names for the limbs, there appear to have been no names given to individual bones. The abdomen was conceived as a basin in which the organs floated. No distinction was made between arteries, veins, ducts, nerves and tendons, which were collectively known as *metou*.

Egyptian physicians took a microcosmic view of the body, drawing certain parallels between its activities and those that occurred in the outer world. According to this view, the *metou* were held to be vessels that maintained and nourished the body in a similar manner to the numerous irrigation channels that nourished the land and provided sustenance for the people. At the centre of this intricate system lay the human heart, which received and distributed the life-giving influences carried through these channels. Both blood and air were believed to circulate to all parts of the body through the *metou*. These channels were said to be particularly extensive around the anus, from which wastes were eliminated from the body.[4]

The Egyptians used emetics, purges and enemas as a matter of course from the time of the Middle Kingdoms. The Greek historian Herodotus records that Egyptians bathed frequently and wore simple, loose clothing. He comments:

> They purge themselves every month, three days in succession seeking to preserve health by emetics and enemas; for they suppose that all diseases to which men are subject proceed from the food they use.[5]

These monthly episodes of ritual cleansing were said to rid the *metou* of decaying intestinal matter. In retrospect, we now know that such practices would have carried great protective value in warding off chronic infestation by the numerous parasites that accompanied the yearly flooding of the Nile. And from a naturopathic perspective, such practices would also have conferred the benefits of regular fasting and elimination on general health.

Such direct methods of interior cleansing have historically been part of a number of healing traditions. The Essene communities of Qumram are said to have made use of enemas for both physical and spiritual healing. Such practices were doubtless carried over from the hygienic rituals of Egypt. The use of clysters and colonic cleansing have also long been part of yogic purification and the regenerative *Rasayana* practices of Ayurvedic medicine.[6]

Within these traditions, colonic cleansing is undertaken in order to remove morbific or stagnant material from the body. Such practices are also consistent with the metaphoric perception of 'the body as temple', which is expressed in both Essene spirituality and the yoga tradition.

In the present day, colonic cleansing finds no place in the methods of biomedicine. Yet contemporary hygienists such as Bernard Jensen have actively promoted and documented the therapeutic value of enemas and colonic irrigation in the treatment of a number of chronic conditions. The intensive use of enemas was also integral to the cancer treatment described by Max Gerson during the 1950s.[7]

Diseases and medicines in ancient Egypt

Much has been learned about the health of the inhabitants of ancient Egypt through examination of the mummified remains preserved in the pyramids and under the desert sands. There is much evidence to suggest that rheumatoid arthritis was relatively common among older Egyptians. The medical papyri reveal that Egyptian physicians had identified this condition and were familiar with its symptoms.

More recent examinations of mummies by pathologists have shown that Egyptians also suffered from arteriosclerosis, smallpox, bubonic plague and Potts disease. Cirrhosis of the liver was a relatively common finding, not surprising, perhaps, in view of the huge amounts of beer and wine said to have been consumed as part of daily life. Many Egyptians also appeared to suffer from trachoma and cataracts.[8] Interestingly, green salts of copper were commonly ground up with animal fats and used as a make-up to highlight the eyes. This is clearly evident in many of the painted images that have survived into the present time. Until recently, copper preparations were used in Western medicine to treat trachoma.

The teeth of pre-Dynastic inhabitants of the older Kingdoms were remarkably free of decay, but appeared to have steadily deteriorated in condition with the increasing use of the softer and more refined foods used by the more affluent newer Kingdoms. It is tempting to draw parallels to the present-day use of processed and refined foods in the Western world which have contributed to the prevalence of the so-called 'diseases of civilisation'.

The castor plant, *Ricinis communis*, was well known in Egypt. The Ebers Papyrus described it as having been 'found in an ancient book concerning the things beneficial to mankind'.[9] The oil pressed from its seeds was used to fuel the numerous lamps that lit up homes at the end of the day. This same oil was used as a purgative in the treatment of constipation and in the monthly cleansing rituals undertaken by many during the later Kingdoms. This particular use of castor oil as a purgative persisted well into the twentieth century. The Ebers Papyrus also records that Egyptian physicians used castor oil as an external application for surface wounds and skin irritations. Castor oil in combination with zinc oxide powder continues to be sold across the counter in many Western pharmacies as an application for skin irritations. The oil itself is known to contain fungistatic constituents.

Yet in more recent times, the castor plant has become a potential source of an influence that is less than 'beneficial to mankind'. Castor seeds are also the source of a potent metabolic poison, ricin, which many in the Western world have begun to fear as a potential weapon in the new armoury of political terrorism. Early in 2003, a number of people were arrested in London under suspicion of producing the lethal toxin ricin from castor seeds.[10] Ricin has been described as 'the third most toxic substance known after plutonium and botulinism'.[11]

Every powerful drug, regardless of its source, will act as a poison when used in high doses. This fact was recognised early by ancient physicians and is an accepted reality in contemporary pharmacology. Such considerations may partially account for the deep-seated suspicion of many within contemporary biomedicine of the use of 'unproven' and 'untested' herbal medicines.

Egyptian physicians of the later Middle Kingdom (approximately 2000 BCE) also knew of the great power of the opium poppy and its sticky exudate, opium. *Papaver* extracts and those of other alkaloid-containing plants may have been used to induce a crude anaesthesia for surgical procedures and the treatment of serious injuries.

The papyri also tell of the use of mouldy bread in the treatment of open wounds. Four thousand years after the Egyptians' use, Alexander Fleming identified the remarkable power hidden within *Penicillium* moulds.

The technicians of ancient Egypt were highly skilled in smelting metals and making glass. Stibnite crystals, antimony trisulphide, were ground finely and mixed with animal fat to produce kohl, a dark and glistening application used to highlight the eyelids. Salts of antimony continue to be used in contemporary Western medicine in the treatment of blood-borne parasitic infestations such as schistosomiasis.

Much attention was given to the treatment of women's conditions in ancient Egypt. Healing substances were introduced into the vagina via suppositories and tampons. Vapour treatments were also commonly used. The papyri record that women would straddle hot stones over which medicinal preparations would be poured. The rising vapours bathed and medicated the genital area.

As Egyptian society began to disintegrate during the time of the newer Kingdoms, much of the medical wisdom acquired through centuries of experience and many of the therapeutic processes and formulae developed by Egyptian physicians was progressively dispersed, along with the numerous artefacts of their civilisation. Many of the individual drugs and approaches to treatment that were more commonly used in Egypt eventually found their way into the medical texts of Dioscorides, Pliny and Galen and, from there, began to exert an influence upon the medical systems of the Greeks, Syrians, Arabs, Persians and Europeans.

Social organisation of Egyptian medicine

The high degree of social organisation that existed in ancient Egypt was matched by that within its healing caste. Writing in the fifth century BCE, Herodotus described the degree of specialisation in Egyptian medicine during the later Kingdoms:

> The art of medicine is thus divided among them: each physician applies himself to one disease only, and not more. All places abound in physicians: some physicians are for the eyes, others for the head, others for the teeth, others for the intestines, and others for internal disorders.[12]

The division of Egyptian medicine into clearly defined specialities was supported by the presence of a number of classes of medical assistants, including nurses, masseurs and midwives. In addition, ancient Egyptian medicine also appears to have been controlled and subsidised by the governing classes.

Deviations from the methods prescribed in the papyri and taught in the *Pir Ankh*, or learning academies, were not only frowned upon, but severely punished on account of 'the law judging that few physicians would ever be wiser than the ways of treatment followed so long, and prescribed originally by the ablest physician'.[13]

Although it is tempting to view the practice of contemporary biomedicine as an unprecedented model of professional organisation, we see within these accounts very clear antecedents of present forms. The differentiation of Egyptian medicine into clearly defined specialities, the near-universal standardisation of treatment methods, and State support of the institution of medicine itself through the subsidy of treatments were not only key elements in the organisation of Egyptian medicine, but have in more recent times become characteristic of Western medicine.

Egyptian physicians were carriers of both sacred knowledge and that gained through many centuries of study and observation of physical injuries and of specific treatments. Many of their methods have survived and continue to have a subtle influence on the practice of medicine today.

There is little doubt that much of early Greek medicine drew strongly from Egyptian sources. In Homeric times, knowledge of both anatomy and therapeutics was far more developed in Egypt than in Greece. However, by the time of Alexander the Great (approximately 320 BCE) a massive reversal had occurred. The formerly potent civilisation of Egypt had become so disorganised and fragmented that young Egyptian physicians had begun to make their way to Greece for further instruction in the art of medicine.

The medicine of Greece

Mediterranean medicine awoke slowly from the dream-state sought in the healing temples of Egypt and early Greece as it turned towards the nascent rationality of Hippocratic times. Doctors no longer waited on the healing dreams of patients, where they hoped to receive divinely inspired guidance for their treatment and management. They began, instead, to more carefully observe their patients' symptoms and to record their findings in meticulous detail. Greek physicians paid increasing attention to both symptom patterns in patients and to the geographical distribution of diseases and epidemics. The sciences of differential diagnosis and epidemiology began to take form.

Greek doctors took a holistic view of their patients, who were seen as the embodiment of natural forces that operated harmoniously in states of health, but that could fall out of balance in disease states. Nature herself was seen as the source of all healing, and the task of the physician was to activate and facilitate the *vis medicatrix naturae*, the restorative or healing power of nature. Dietary and sanitary principles were to become strong elements in the emergent therapeutics of Greece.

The seventy books of the Hippocratic Collection reflect both the depth and detail embodied in Greek medicine at that time. But a knowledge of the body, in terms of the anatomy and physiology that we take for granted today, had yet to fully develop.

Awakenings

Early Greek medicine developed around a complex mythology. The Greeks' chief god of healing was the great Apollo. When angered by the deeds of humans, he would shoot arrows into the earth and strike down entire communities with epidemics of plague and sickness. Apollo was equally capable of protecting against these same onslaughts and of healing the afflicted. He was physician to the gods of Olympus.

The Greek physician Asklepios is said to have been born of a union between Apollo and the beautiful maiden Coronis. While yet a young man, Asklepios was drawn to the healing arts, and after qualifying as a physician he gained renown as a powerful healer. His two daughters, Hygeia and Panacea, were to lend their names to profoundly enduring understandings which remain part of the broader language of healing even today.

The great healing successes of Asklepios angered Pluto, the god of the underworld, who complained that the treatments of Asklepios were keeping people alive too long and were denying Hades its rightful number of souls. He called on his brother Zeus, lord of the gods, to intervene. Asklepios was promptly struck down by a bolt of lightning.

Asklepios thereby took his own place among the gods of healing. Those who followed in his tradition set up an organised guild of doctor-priests, the *Asklepiads*, who sought his intervention in the healing of patients through invocation and worship. Over 300 sanctuaries of healing dedicated to Asklepios were built throughout Greece, the first being built around 700 BCE. The most impressive were those of Cos, Epidaurus, Cnidus and Pergamos. These early hospitals were often situated near forest springs and mountain streams, places that not only provided water in abundance but which were also said to attract great healing energies.

The healing temples of Asklepios

The seeds of rationality present in early Greek medicine sprouted from a magical consciousness and were watered by a powerful and complex mythology. In the healing temples of Asklepios, the attention of the doctor-priests was directed more to the images that emerged in the dreams of patients than to their bodily signs and symptoms. The study of the role of dreams in patients' lives was to persist, and was later incorporated into Hippocratic medicine.

Patients would be welcomed into the *Asklepieia*, or temples of healing, by the Asklepiads, who would recount stories of the remarkable healings that had occurred there. There would then follow a period of prayer and sacred ceremony. Images and records of successful healings surrounded new patients; these were carved into the walls and pillars of the temple itself, and were displayed in the numerous figurines that had been offered as gifts by grateful patients.

New arrivals would bathe in the healing mineral springs around which many of the temples were built, and would be massaged with fragrant oils. They would then make their way to the central *abaton*, or incubation chamber, where they would sleep and await the visitation of a healing guide in a dream. The dreams of patients were heard by their Asklepiad attendants, who would then devise a treatment based on these nocturnal intimations. Patients who were cured of their condition would often present the temple with a gift in the form of an effigy, crafted in wax, stone or precious metal, of the diseased body part which had been healed. Numerous such votive offerings have been recovered from these ancient hospital/temples by archaeologists.

Although it may be tempting to dismiss such stories as being based on myth and superstition, they nonetheless point towards a dimension of healing with which biomedicine remains largely unfamiliar and mildly uncomfortable. We continue to hear echoes of such healing stories as those told on the temple walls of Epidaurus in the experiences of many who undertake healing pilgrimages to such places as Lourdes and Medjugorje today.

Empedocles of Agrigentum

The philosopher Empedocles lived during the fifth century BCE. Six hundred years after his death, he was described by the Greek physician Galen as the founder of the science of medicine in Italy. Empedocles is also remembered as a mystic and poet. His teachings regarding the four elements had a profound influence on both philosophy and medicine in ancient Greece. They were to remain a major force in European medicine for the following two thousand years.

Empedocles taught that the world is formed and sustained by the elemental qualities of earth, air, fire and water. He framed many of his teachings about the phenomenal world in poetic terms:

> Hear first the four roots of all things:
> Bright Zeus [fire], life-giving Hera (air),
> And Aidoneus (earth), and Nestis [water]
> Who moistens the springs of men with her tears.[14]

This fragment represents the first coherent expression of the doctrine of the four elements. Greek doctors and philosophers readily took up this notion in their quest to understand and interpret the world. Both Plato and Aristotle were familiar with the works of Empedocles.

In addition to his contributions to early philosophy and medicine, Empedocles also took on a number of major engineering projects that were to benefit the health of those of his home town and its surroundings. He is credited with halting an epidemic of malaria in Agrigentum, in Sicily, by draining the surrounding swamplands. For this, Empedocles was publicly hailed as a great healer. This extraordinary feat of urban sanitation was later to be repeated by Luigi Cornaro, an Italian architect and writer on the art of longevity, who similarly drained the fetid swamps of his home city of Venice at the turn of the Renaissance.

The genius of Empedocles oversaw another feat of engineering which resulted in a remarkable easing of the climatic condition of Agrigentum. In a project equal to the major engineering works of Egypt, a large cleft in a nearby mountainside was blocked off and the scorching winds of the sirocco, blowing from the deserts of North Africa, were thereby deflected.

Empedocles' more enduring gift to posterity, however, was the doctrine of the four elements. Air, earth, fire and water were identified with the qualities of heat, cold, dryness and moisture. The human body and its expressions in health and disease were interpreted in similar terms. Air was seen as hot and moist and was related to blood and the sanguine temperament. The earth principle was said to be cold and dry and associated with phlegmatic tendencies. Fire was hot and dry and related to the yellow bile which inflamed choleric temperaments and jaundiced skin when in excess. And the element of water was seen as cold and moist and reflected in black bile and a tendency to melancholy.

Greek physicians based their clinical interpretations on this system in their attempt to understand human sickness and their pursuit of appropriate treatments. This elemental, or humoral, paradigm was to dominate European therapeutics for a period of nearly two thousand years, until the iconoclastic reforms of Paracelsus began to fracture the dogmatism embedded in sixteenth-century European medicine.

The medicine taught by Galen and that developed by Arab physicians were both built upon this elemental system. Medicinal substances were classified according to the suggested preponderance of each of these four elemental influences. According to this system, for example, cardamoms were said to be warm in the first degree, cold by one half a degree, dry in the first degree and so on. Patients' diseases would be similarly classified. The task of the doctor was to devise appropriate treatments and medicinal formulations in order to augment deficient qualities, and to diminish overactive qualities. This humoral or qualitative approach to diagnosis and treatment continues to influence the traditional medicines of both India and China.

Hippocrates of Cos

Hippocrates was born around 460 BCE and continues to be identified as the great exemplar of the principles and ethical ideals of early Greek medicine. He received his first instructions from his father, who was an Asklepiad. As a young man, Hippocrates studied in Athens and then travelled widely, learning and practising in the cities of Thrace, Thessaly and Macedonia. The medical writings with which he has become identified were a revolutionary departure from the mythical and mystical leanings of the medicine of Egypt and the later Asklepiad healing temples.

The Hippocratic writings brought together into a systematic framework the collective knowledge of the main Greek schools of medicine. Much of Hippocratic doctrine was built upon the humoral pathology of the time. The unique contribution of Hippocrates, however, was expressed in his call for physicians to observe their patients more attentively, to record their signs and symptoms in detail, and to live according to the highest moral and ethical principles.

Hippocratic doctors paid close attention to such details as facial appearance, pulse, temperature, respiration, quality of urine, faeces and sputum, and movements of the body, as the following clinical history, recorded some two and a half thousand years ago, demonstrates:

> Seventh case: A woman at the house of Aristion with sore throat, which began from the tongue; speech indistinct, tongue red and becoming parched. First day, she felt chilly, and was then feverish. Third day, a rigor, and acute fever; a reddish hard oedema on both sides of the neck and chest; extremities cold and livid; respiration laboured; fluids returned through the nose; could not drink; constipation and suppression of urine. Fourth day, all symptoms grew worse. Fifth day, the patient died.[15]

The detail expressed in this observation and in many others signals the origins of an analytical sensitivity that has since become the hallmark of contemporary scientific medicine.

The writings identified with Hippocrates also reveal a clear understanding of the nature and treatment of bone fractures and dislocations. Much of the valuable experience of many generations of Egyptian doctors was assimilated by early Greek medicine.

The Hippocratic writings advise against the use of ointments and greasy dressings in the treatment of open wounds, recommending only clean water or wine to wash affected areas, and the occasional use of astringent plant washes to promote knitting of the wound edges. For the treatment of infected and suppurating wounds, most Greek doctors used only boiled water. It was also recommended that their own hands and fingernails be well cleaned before treating open wounds.

It is an extraordinary fact that what we now consider to be common sense, expressed in such medical writings over two thousand years ago, was lost to the profession for so long. The Austrian doctor Ignaz Semmelweis was laughed out of his profession when he insisted in 1857 that fewer women would die in childbirth in the obstetric wards of Viennese hospitals if doctors and medical students simply washed their hands after dissecting cadavers in the hospital basement before attending the labour ward. Maddened by the hostility and criticism of his colleagues, Semmelweis was committed to an asylum, where he died in 1865. Change appears to come slowly in many areas of medicine.

Although Hippocratic medicine made use of many powerful plant-based medicines, its primary aim in treatment was to support natural healing forces through the provision of rest, fresh air, good diet, and through such methods as purging and emesis. Barley gruel was commonly used in digestive disturbances, and barley water, honey and water, honey and vinegar, massage and water treatments were also widely prescribed.[16] Doctors of the time made use of black hellebore (*Helleborus niger*) as a purging agent, and white hellebore (*Veratrum album*) as an emetic. Unlike the Egyptians, who used a huge range of medicinal substances, Greek doctors tended to favour the use of a smaller number of highly potent plant medicines whose effects were readily visible and often dramatic.

In Hippocratic medicine, the primary focus of the doctor was on the patient and on their symptoms. The view of disease as an invasion by noxious and demonic forces that characterised earlier Egyptian medicine was overshadowed by a view of disease as an expression of the body's struggle to eliminate 'morbid materials' through its natural self-healing tendency.

Theophrastus of Eresus

Hippocrates died at around 70 years of age. At around that time, the young Aristotle was just beginning his studies in medicine under the direction of Asklepiad teachers. Aristotle was later to pursue studies in philosophy under Plato. Although Aristotle is remembered as one of the great analytical philosophers of antiquity, he also gave to Greek medicine an enduring impetus towards the newly developing disciplines of botany, zoology, comparative anatomy, embryology and physiology. His historical influence lives on in the commitment of contemporary biomedicine to a profoundly analytic epistemology of the body and disease.

Theophrastus of Eresus (c. 370–286 BCE) was considered by Aristotle to be his finest student. Before his death, Aristotle bequeathed all his books and his botanic gardens to Theophrastus, made him guardian of his children and designated him successor of his school.

Theophrastus had learnt well from his master. He was among the first to gather and collate all the known information on plants and their uses. His *De Historia Plantarum*, written in ten books, contains descriptions of some 500 plants, many of which were used as medicines at the time. In accordance with the highly analytical approach of his teacher Aristotle, he described the various plant structures, from roots to fruits, studied seed development in plants, and identified differences between monocotyledons and dicotyledons. Theophrastus attempted to collect and summarise all the available knowledge of his time regarding the medicinal properties of plants. His sources ranged from the writings of Homer to the reports of Mediterranean travellers about the arrow poisons used by African tribes.

In the *De Historia Plantarum*, Theophrastus laid the foundations for a new method of investigation and documentation that culminated four centuries later in the *De Materia Medica* of Pedanius Dioscorides. The superbly organised and exhaustive collections of information concerning substances used as medicines gathered by Theophrastus and Dioscorides were to become the primary sources of a stable pharmacopoeia that was used by both European and Arabic doctors until a little over one hundred years ago.

The enduring legacy

The purpose of studying the past is to illuminate the present. Even though our collective memory may be limited to what is directly before us, it is important to understand that the medicine practised in the West today continues to be subtly influenced by the notions and ideas that upheld earlier practices. We may pride ourselves on our degree of mastery in such areas as anatomy, pathophysiology, pharmacology and surgery, yet the true measure of health resides in more than the health of our bodies. We each live an inner life, are moved by hopes and fears, participate in social realities, and inhabit a world of conflicting interests.

The medical practices of Egypt and Greece helped lay the foundations for an historic project that will continue for as long as humanity inhabits the earth. Egyptian and Greek physicians each made use of substances they believed would enable health to be regained in times of sickness. This approach, though radically transformed in terms of the substances used, continues to form the basis of contemporary pharmaceutics. During the intervening centuries, knowledge of many of these substances has been quietly transmitted both through folkloric use and the herbal texts that continue to form the basis for the practice of contemporary herbal medicine.

These medicines, produced in the great laboratory of nature, will always be available to us as long as we retain our connection with the earth and the natural cycles that govern plant growth and reproduction.

Both Egypt and Greece have also provided us with templates for a trustful therapeutics that honours the capacity of living systems for regeneration and self-healing. The hygienist principles reflected in the monthly cleansing rituals of later Egypt, and the conservative therapeutics of Hippocratic physicians who made use of such methods as rest, exercise and careful attention to diet, remain relevant to healing though they may not figure prominently in the methods of biomedicine.

The hieratic, or priestly, side of physicianship was strongly evident in both the healing rituals and invocations used by Egyptian physicians and in the intention of those who ministered in the healing temples of Isis and, later, Asklepios. This form of psychosomatic medicine cannot be lightly brushed off as a useless artefact of more superstitious times. Human nature will always be influenced for better or worse by hopes and aspirations, by dreams and expectations. This priestly aspect of physicianship has, perhaps, been overshadowed by the present Western style, based as it is upon high rationality and the use of powerful technologies, yet will always remain available as a source of both healing and comfort.

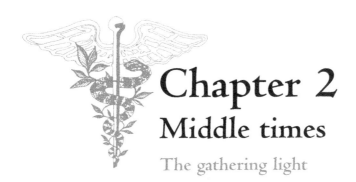

Chapter 2
Middle times
The gathering light

Nature is the physician, not you; from her you take your orders, not from yourself; she composes, not you.

Paracelsus, c. 1530[1]

The greater physicians of the past, reasoning from what seem to us to be very faulty premises, somehow got their patients well, otherwise they would have had no clientele or following. The thing is to ascertain, if possible, just how they did it.

Fielding Garrison, 1929[2]

The new Hippocratic medicine established the central importance of detailed observation and analytical thought in the quest to understand health and disease. Yet the realisation of that process was to remain dormant for many generations. Until the time of the Renaissance, medical knowledge held strongly to the humoral medicine taught by Galen in the second century CE, and refined by Avicenna in the eleventh century. Both Galen and Avicenna were deemed infallible in their judgements. A truly physiological knowledge of the body and its diseases was to remain elusive for more than two thousand years.

Many ancient medical texts were preserved and copied by hand by Catholic monks and Arab scholars until the development of the printing press in the fifteenth century. This led to an unprecedented release of works that had previously been in the possession of libraries and private collections.

As knowledge began to disseminate more widely, and as earlier prohibitions on the study of human anatomy slowly lifted, the theories of humoral medicine and early descriptions of the body and its functions became increasingly difficult to reconcile with the new anatomical observations. Andreas Vesalius charted this new terrain in his *De Humani Corporis Fabrica*, published in 1543. William Harvey followed soon after and blew apart the hallowed notions of millennia with his revelation that blood circulated continuously throughout the body.

The European Renaissance gave rise to powerful new technologies and to new ways of investigating the phenomenal world. Ancient paradigms that had shaped the intellectual life of Europe for centuries were challenged by knowledge that told a new story about the nature of life and the universe. The development of the telescope enabled Kepler, Copernicus and Galileo to show beyond doubt that the earth was not the centre of the universe. The development of microscopes soon after revealed the existence of totally unexpected miniature worlds.

Such discoveries began to shake the fixed structures in European culture. The Catholic church actively opposed the intrusion of such new knowledge, as it directly challenged its own authority by presenting differing views of life and the world to its own. The European medical establishment itself was also slow to change, preferring to hold on to the ancient ways described in Greek and Arabic texts.

The two thousand years that elapsed between the Hippocratic awakening and the next major turning that occurred during the Renaissance was, in terms of the development of medicine, one of relative stability and consolidation. This was, perhaps, the calm before the storm. Yet during that time, there arose a number of significant movements that were to exert their own influence on European medicine.

Pedanius Dioscorides

The meticulous attention to detail that characterised the approach of the early Hippocratic physicians was new to both medicine and the study of natural phenomena. This marked a turning point in Western consciousness, as philosopher-scientists began to focus less upon interiority and conjecture, and to more strongly direct their attention to the natural world. This new philosophical approach was given early impetus by Aristotle in the fourth century BCE, and was applied systematically to a study of the plant kingdom by his successor, Theophrastus.

Pedanius Dioscorides was born in Greece in the early part of the first century CE and became one of the greatest compilers of natural medicines and their uses in history. He is universally honoured, even today, in numerous published works on plant medicines. On completing his medical studies, Dioscorides travelled widely throughout the known world in order to increase his knowledge of the substances used as medicines. He visited 38 provinces, cities and mountains in Asia Minor (present-day Turkey), the Greek mainland, Egypt, Syria and Italy. He was also familiar with parts of Arabia, Spain, Africa, Persia, India and Armenia. Dioscorides gained his knowledge of medicinal substances by observing them in their natural habitats, and through discussions with the healers and inhabitants of the places he visited.[3]

Following the approach laid down by Aristotle and Theophrastus, Dioscorides described in great detail the medicinal properties of over 1000 natural products, of which over 600 were plants. This compilation gathered together all the knowledge of medicinal plants available in the Mediterranean at the time. Dioscorides described the actions of medicines in physiological, rather than humoral, terms. He was more interested in their specific effects than in their theoretical attributes. He gave little, if any, attention to their magical or non-medical uses.

His resultant text, *De Materia Medica*, became the standard pharmacopoeia of the time and was used widely in the Greek, Arabic and European schools of medicine. American historian John Riddle described the influence of Dioscorides in the following terms:

> For the sixteen hundred years of the modern era, the knowledge of medi-cines came more from the prodigious search effort of one man, Dioscorides (fl. ca. A.D. 40–80), than from any other person. While he may not have been the first to discover most of the usages, he industriously collected them from various lands, codified the data, and organized it in a clear, concise, and rational fashion. For this reason, he became the chief author-ity on pharmacy and one of the principal ones on medicine.[4]

The compiling of *De Materia Medica* was an extraordinary undertaking. Apart from its size and scope, it reflected a surprisingly modern understanding of the action of medicines. Dioscorides distanced himself from the academic debates and theorising that characterised much of the Greek medicine of the time. He did not buy into the prevailing humoral theories of the time. In this regard, he took his lead from Celsus, a contemporary Roman physician who described medicinal plants in terms of their actions on the human body rather than their humoral attributes.

In the preface to *De Materia Medica*, Dioscorides explicitly rejected the common practice of arranging his subject matter either alphabetically, or according to the humoral system of classification commonly used at that time. Instead, he grouped his medicines according to their actions as cathartic, emetic, narcotic, expectorant, vulnerary, and so on. He thereby anticipated by some 1500 years the notion that plants and other medicinal agents contained classes of pharmacologically active constituents that were responsible for their particular effects on the body.

Each plant is painstakingly detailed in individual chapters. Each chapter includes the name of the plant and a full botanical description, its painted image, its various habitats, its pharmacological properties or types of action, medicinal uses, side effects, quantities and dosage, harvesting, preparation and storage instructions, adulteration and methods of detection, and the specific geographical locations where the plants occurred naturally.

The monumental *De Materia Medica* marked the emergence of pharmacology as a science and therapeutic discipline. It soon took its place as one of the leading medical texts in Europe, the Middle East and Asia Minor. The work of Dioscorides remains largely unknown to practitioners of biomedicine. Yet practitioners of contemporary herbal medicine throughout the world continue to make use of many of the medicines described in his epochal text.

Galen of Pergamon

Of greater influence on the subsequent course of both Islamic and European medicine was the work of the prolific writer and physician Galen. Galen was born in Pergamon around 130 CE. His father, the well-connected Nikon, was the king's architect. He took charge of his son's education from an early age and groomed him for a life in politics. Galen began studies in mathematics, philosophy and science when he was fourteen years of age. His father was unexpectedly visited in a dream by Asklepios, who told him that his son was fated for a future in medicine. Old Nikon immediately introduced his son to the circle of physicians associated with the Asklepion, the healing sanctuary in Pergamon, and Galen spent the next four years in their company engaged in the study of medicine.

From the outset, Galen was attracted to the works of the Hippocratic school and to the study of anatomy. This passion was to remain with him all his days. His father died unexpectedly in 148 or 149 CE, leaving him in possession of great wealth and near total freedom at the age of 20. Galen spent the following ten years in further medical studies at the schools of Smyrna, Corinth and Alexandria. Even during those early years he wrote prolifically on anatomy and physiology.

Galen returned to his native Pergamon when in his late twenties as an established writer and physician. Soon after he was appointed physician to the gladiators of the city. This enabled him to further his knowledge of anatomy and surgery, as many of those in his charge suffered from injuries inflicted by heavy swords and other weapons. As physician to the gladiators, Galen organised their dietary patterns along Hippocratic lines in order to best maintain their physical fitness. He also had charge of a large dispensary and hospital-like infirmary where the more seriously wounded were treated.[5]

During his early thirties, Galen left Pergamon for Rome where he was to spend most of the rest of his life. He moved in powerful circles and within a short time was appointed physician to the emperor, Marcus Aurelius. His time in Rome established him as an important writer in the fields of medicine, logic and philosophy. Galen's medical writings encompassed virtually the entirety of existing medical thought and practice of the time, and also included his own unique contributions in the fields of anatomy, physiology and therapeutics. Included in his writings were several commentaries on the Hippocratic texts.

Galen brought a mix of attentive observation and philosophical interpretation to his method. The consequence was a paradoxical blend of astute physiological insight and the speculative dogma that was to dominate the practice of European medicine for many centuries. He ascertained that blood rather then air, as had earlier been believed, moved through the arteries. And he came close to discovering the circulation of the blood, recognising that the heart served to pump blood through those arteries. Yet he never made the full connection, believing that blood moved through the body like the tide, ebbing and flowing consecutively. A further 1500 years were to elapse before Harvey corrected his mistaken notions. He also held that the blood itself was produced by the liver, passed from the right to the left side of the heart through a series of fine pores in the septum or dividing wall, and was filtered by the brain, with impurities being discharged in the form of phlegm, saliva, tears and sweat.

Galen did much to popularise and reinforce the hygienic teachings of Hippocrates, yet believed that infection was a normal and necessary part of the healing of wounds, even describing pus formation as *bonum et laudabile*, or 'good and praiseworthy'.[6] It took a further 1400 years before Paracelsus enjoined European physicians to work with clean hands and to wash open wounds with fresh water or wine in the manner of the Hippocratic teachings.

Galen extended the prevailing humoral theories of physiology inherited from Hippocratic physicians. He was the first to relate the individual humours of blood, phlegm, yellow bile and black bile that were used to interpret the nature of disease, to human temperament and psychology. He consequently classified individuals according to the four personality types of sanguine, phlegmatic, choleric and melancholic.

In his own life and work, Galen attained both wealth and fame. He believed himself to be the greatest living authority on medicine at the time, and ferociously denounced those who did not accept his views. History accorded him his desired status. Galen's writings were considered by both

European and Arab physicians to be an infallible source of medical knowledge for well over a thousand years.

His hold on the mind of European medicine was, however, symbolically loosened when the *Kanun* of Avicenna, based largely on Galen's humoral system, was thrown by Paracelsus into a student bonfire at the University of Basle in 1527. Sixteen years later, Andreas Vesalius published his own anatomical findings based upon many years of human dissection. In it, he made over 200 corrections to Galen's anatomical observations. Predictably, both Paracelsus and Vesalius were fiercely denounced by many of their peers as heretics.

Galen's contribution provided an enduring framework for both medical theory and practice for many centuries. Although he provided a number of unique insights, his influence also contributed to a fixation of medical thinking until the reforms associated with Renaissance times. But adherence to dogma was not the exclusive domain of the profession of medicine. This tendency appeared to be universal in all groups that exercised power in any form, from the church down.

The hidden currents

One often encounters the term *Graeco-Arabic* in discussions of the medicine of pre-Renaissance times. This points to the subtle yet highly influential role of Arabic scholars and physicians in the transmission of the medical knowledge that eventually took firm root within Europe. Arab physicians were largely responsible for the translation and preservation of many of the ancient Greek medical texts. The Greek original was often preserved along with the Arabic translations of such works. This enabled future generations of European scholars to undertake their own translations from the original Greek script.

Arabic culture flourished over a three-century period from the mid-600s until the end of the first millennium CE. The Islamic expansion into Spain by the mid-700s brought with it an influx of scholars and physicians who created a powerful cultural and intellectual nucleus that was to have a strong influence on European thought in subsequent centuries.

Arabic scholars actively sought out the texts of medicine and philosophy produced by Greek and Roman writers. Physicians were particularly drawn to the works of Aristotle, Hippocrates, Dioscorides and Galen, and their works were widely reproduced and translated. In fact, some of the Greek texts would have been completely lost to history were it not for surviving Arabic translations.[7]

Due to the prohibition of anatomical investigations by the laws of the Koran, Arab physicians cleaved strongly to the humoral medicine of Galen.

They were, however, free to develop and extend their knowledge of pharmaceutics and pharmacology. This not only ensured the continuing influence of the works of Theophrastus and Dioscorides, but enabled the art of medicinal chemistry to develop in new directions.

Islamic medicine found its strongest expression in the works of two Persian physicians, Rhazes and Avicenna. Rhazes was born around 850 CE, while Avicenna was born over a century later, around 980 CE. Both were prolific writers and produced encyclopedic compilations of the medical knowledge of their day. Avicenna in particular had a strong influence on both Islamic and European medicine through his *El Kanun*, or 'Canon of Medicine', that 'soon supplanted in the West the works of the Greeks and, until the time of the humanists, served as the most important textbook for physicians'.[8] Much of Avicenna's *Kanun* consisted of poetic interpretations of the humoral medicine of Galen.

Arabic scholars slowly made their way from Spain into other European theatres, bringing with them their texts and translations. Two major centres of learning were to benefit significantly from their influence: the school of Montpellier in France, and that of Salerno in Italy. Both were to become renowned for their contributions to the development of European medicine.

Salerno

University training in medicine only became established in the early centuries of the second millennium. The first European school of medicine was in Salerno, then an old Doric colony near Naples, which was founded around 1000 CE. Salerno was directed, though not controlled, by the Catholic church, and its teachers included both priests and secular scholars.

The first group of teachers at Salerno was remarkably eclectic for the times, and included Greek, Jewish, Arab and Latin scholars. Both men and women were represented in this group. And both women and Jews were welcomed as students at Salerno, which further reflected an extraordinary liberalism for the times. Such revolutionary developments anticipated the intellectual freedoms that would eventually come to characterise academic education in the West, though it would take many centuries for this to be fully realised.

The school of medicine at Salerno initially taught the Galenic medicine favoured by Arab physicians. As more of the texts brought by Arabic scholars began to be translated into Latin, the school increasingly moved in the direction of the Hippocratic teachings, and within a relatively short time Salerno became a focus for the renewal of Hippocratic ideas and ideals. The

Hippocratic spirit so dominated the school that it eventually became known as the *Civitas Hippocratica*, or society of Hippocrates.

Among the teachers at Salerno was Trotula of Ruggiero, a renowned physician and obstetrician. She wrote a number of works on obstetrics and gynaecology that became standard texts in European universities for several centuries. Trotula is remembered as the first female professor of medicine in recorded history. She favoured a Hippocratic style of medicine and encouraged attention to diet, regular physical activity and cleanliness in matters of personal hygiene.[9] Her presence within the European medical academy was, however, but a momentary illumination that soon after faded for many centuries, as both university and medical education became increasingly male dominated.

The school at Salerno was also the first European university whose graduates were endorsed and recognised by the State. In 1140 CE, King Roger II of Sicily decreed that formal qualifications were necessary for the practice of medicine. Prospective doctors were required to pass examinations set by the faculty at Salerno. This development was furthered in 1224 CE by his grandson, King Frederick II, who ruled that candidates for qualification as doctors of medicine needed to have completed five years of formal medical studies and undertaken a further year in supervised practise before being eligible to attend examinations at Salerno.

These developments placed medicine on a strong academic footing that was to be sustained, in one way or another, into the present time. This situation also created an early divide between the 'schoolmen' and 'lay' practitioners of medicine. University-trained physicians tended to serve the wealthy, particularly in urban environments, while those who could not afford treatments were attended by monastic orders, itinerate healers and those within their own communities who had knowledge of medicinal substances and traditional ways of healing.

The tension between a sanctioned and highly educated professional medical elite and healers whose knowledge has been acquired by other means is perhaps a perennial reality. That tension has reappeared most recently in the periodic contentions that characterised relations between practitioners of biomedicine and practitioners of alternative and complementary medicine during the latter decades of the twentieth century.

The new academies

Human dissection was not undertaken at Salerno due to the influence of Islamic teachers and an ecclesiastical aversion to interference with corpses. Early anatomical studies at Salerno tended to follow the pattern established by Galen, and depended mainly upon the dissection of animals.

The first medical school to inaugurate human dissection as part of its program was that at Bologna. The Catholic University of Bologna began to teach medicine during the twelfth century. Although the school had a strong Galenic orientation, it broke with earlier conventions and introduced human dissection soon after being established.

Anatomy teacher Mondino de Luzzi wrote the first known treatise on dissection while at Bologna in 1316. Early editions were copied by hand until the first printed editions became available in 1487. Despite its numerous errors, Mondino's text became the main source of anatomical knowledge in European medical schools until Vesalius published his revolutionary *De Humanis Corpora Fabrica* in 1543.

King Frederick II, who had set the standards for medical education at Salerno in 1224, clearly had an active interest in higher education. He was instrumental in setting up yet another university at Padua in 1222. Many of the teachers from Bologna defected to Padua and its reputation grew rapidly. Although Mondino's anatomical work at Bologna had established a clear precedent, human dissection was not taught in Padua until 1341, twenty-five years after Mondino wrote his first treatise. Yet Padua would eventually become the new centre of anatomical studies that, in time, completely transformed the knowledge base of medicine.

It was at Padua that Andreas Vesalius was to take up the position of lecturer in anatomy in 1539. He was succeeded by his assistant, Realdo Colombo, in 1546. Realdo in turn passed the torch on to Gabriele Fallopio, who is remembered for his studies of the female reproductive system and after whom the fallopian tubes are named. Fallopio was succeeded by Gironamo Fabrizio, who studied the valvular structures within veins. Englishman William Harvey undertook his medical studies at Padua, and was taught anatomy by Fabrizio. After graduating from Padua, Harvey took up a position as lecturer in anatomy at the College of Physicians in London. He further extended Fabrizio's earlier studies of the blood and circulatory system, and in 1628 published his revolutionary findings detailing the circulation of blood through the body. Like Vesalius, from whose direct lineage he had emerged, Harvey was also condemned and opposed by many of his colleagues for presenting views that challenged the authority of Galen.[10]

The new knowledge that erupted throughout Europe in all fields of human endeavour created a turbulence that severely shook the established order. The discoveries of the telescope and the microscope had each extended human vision into unprecedented realms. The limits of the world itself were similarly extended when Christopher Columbus confirmed that the earth was a massive sphere that wheeled through space. The formerly sacrosanct power of the Catholic church began to be challenged simultaneously on numerous fronts. Medicine itself was no exception to the assault of the times. The ancient knowledge that had served physicians so well was increasingly questioned. Many faltering attempts were made to prop up the established structures, but the force of truth, the power of direct experience over dogma, and the currents of change that were transforming human consciousness at the time could not be resisted indefinitely. It was at this critical time that Paracelsus appeared on the scene.

Paracelsus of Einseideln

Paracelsus was born Phillippus Aureolus Theophrastus Bombastus von Hohenheim in 1493, one year after Columbus discovered the new world. In many ways he went on to embody the turmoil of his times. Paracelsus identified completely with the mission of medicine, at various times describing himself as its monarch. He received an early grounding in the knowledge of the times through the influence of his physician father, and of his early teachers, many of whom were high clerics with deep interests in alchemy, theology and the new technologies.

Having lost his mother while still a boy, he learnt to rough it from a young age as he travelled with his father. Paracelsus was on the move for most of his life, resting only long enough in any one place to stir up a storm among the local medical and municipal authorities before hastily making his way again. He held university training in little regard, despite having studied at the Universities of Vienna and Ferrara and visiting a number of others on his travels. Throughout his relatively short life, Paracelsus championed the importance of direct experience over the books and dogma that ruled the day. He commented:

> Not all things the physician must know are taught in the academies. Now and then he must turn to old women, to Tartars who are called gypsies, to itinerant magicians, to elderly country folk and many others who are frequently held in contempt. From them he will gather his knowledge since these people have more understanding of such things than all the high colleges.[11]

Paracelsus was a contradictory character who seemed to evoke, both during his life and posthumously, either great admiration or deep contempt. Yet he made a lasting impression upon his own times and remains a source of inspiration for many, even today.

Paracelsus was particularly drawn to one of his teachers at Ferrara, Nicolo Leoniceno. Leoniceno had translated a number of the Greek medical authors and instilled in his young student a love of Hippocrates and a fascination with the newly translated ideas of the Roman physician Celsus. Leoniceno was strongly critical of the dogmatic teachings of Avicenna, whose *Kanun* was at that time universally taught in European schools of medicine.

The young Paracelsus struggled to reconcile the alchemical teachings of his Benedictine mentors with a newly emerging understanding of how plant medicines performed their healing work. Leoniceno's view of pharmacology was based more on the approach of Celsus and Dioscorides than that of Galen and Avicenna.

Neither Celsus nor Dioscorides described medicinally active substances according to the prevailing humoral doctrine, but rather classified the medicines of their time according to their specific activity or 'virtue'. Celsus described medicines as purgatives, diaphoretics, diuretics, emetics, narcotics and so on. Paracelsus was immediately attracted to this new interpretation, so different from Galen's humoral understanding.

On graduating from Ferrara late in 1515 at the age of 22, he took on the name *Para*celsus in acknowledgement of the influence of the ideas of Celsus on his own development. This was no arrogant claim that he was 'greater than Celsus'; by taking on this name, he sealed a commitment to deepening his understanding of how medicinally active substances exerted their influence.

In describing the action of medicinal substances, he spoke of the *arcana* within medicines that enabled them to do their work. These arcana were hidden principles that we now know to be the specific active chemical constituents within medicines. He asked questions that could not be answered by the medicine of the time:

> It does not matter that rhubarb is a purgative. The question is: What is it that purges? Not the answer, rhubarb purges; but the answer: What is the *corpus* that purges? Names do not have virtues. Substances do.[12]

Paracelsus remained equally conscious of the need to understand the luminous and spiritual aspects of reality. Throughout his writings, he constantly referred to 'the light of nature'.

On completing his formal medical studies, Paracelsus travelled continuously for ten years, consolidating his knowledge of medicine. Like many of his young colleagues, he spent some time as an army doctor. His travels with the military brought him into contact with the epidemics of syphilis that were searing numerous cities in Italy and France, and he had many opportunities to observe how different communities dealt with conditions that had never been described before.

Paracelsus was present in Moscow during the siege of the Tartar tribesmen in 1520. His status as a physician assured his freedom in exchange for his skills and services. He was welcomed as a peer by the Tartar shamans, who regarded the work of healers as sacred. Tartar medicine men attributed much of their power and influence to the spirits of departed ancestors and mentors. Paracelsus was later to write extensively on the many spiritual forces that operate in the natural world.

He returned to his native Switzerland in the mid-1520s and soon gained a reputation as a vocal and energetic physician. He was unexpectedly called to the house of Johannes Froben, a wealthy and influential publisher in Basel who had earlier suffered a stroke that had left him partially paralysed. One of his legs had become severely infected and was no longer responding to treatment. His physicians had advised that his leg needed to be amputated. Froben called for the newly arrived doctor. Within a few days, the infection had resolved and old Froben began to walk freely again.

The humanist scholar Erasmus of Rotterdam, a close friend of Froben, happened to be visiting him at the time. Erasmus saw for himself the remarkable recovery brought about by the treatment of the rough and fiery young man who had just arrived on the scene. And young Paracelsus suddenly found himself in the presence of a man whose work he had long admired. Though of totally different natures, they enjoyed many discussions. After Froben's cure, Erasmus wrote to Paracelsus:

> I cannot offer any compensation adequate to your art, but I promise to bear gratitude toward you. You have brought back from hell Froben, who is my other half. If you restore my health too, you will give us back to each other. Let fortune retain you in Basel.[13]

Erasmus and his circle of friends opened a few doors in order to help such fortune along. Paracelsus was soon offered the post of town physician and a professorship in the faculty of medicine at the University of Basel. But his patrons had sorely underestimated the passion of their new charge.

Paracelsus' appointment was largely ignored by the medical faculty itself. He claimed his new freedom as an opportunity to throw open the doors of academic medicine. On 5 June 1527, he placed a copy of his new curriculum on the announcement board of the university. In it, he proclaimed his program for the reform of medicine:

> It seems imperative to bring medicine back to its original laudable state, and, aside from striving to cleanse it of the dregs left by the barbarians, to purify it of the most serious errors. Not according to the rules of the ancients, but solely according to those which we have found proved by the nature of things through practice and experience . . .
>
> It is not title and eloquence, nor the knowledge of languages, nor the reading of many books, however ornamental, that are the requirements of

a physician, but the deepest knowledge of things themselves and of nature's secrets, and this knowledge outweighs all else.[14]

Shortly after taking up his new position, Paracelsus ceremoniously cast the *Kanun* of Avicenna into the flames at a large student bonfire, so that 'all this misery may go in the air with the smoke'.[15] This act of heresy enraged the faculty, and they denied him further access to his lecture theatre in the university grounds. He took his classes elsewhere.

In his role as town physician, Paracelsus also made many enemies. He vigorously attacked the profit-sharing 'arrangement' between the physicians and the apothecaries of Basel. Before long, Paracelsus had managed not only to alienate the medical faculty, but most of the doctors and pharmacists in Basel as well.

The crunch finally came when he sued a wealthy churchman, Cornelius von Lichtenfels, for recovery of unpaid fees. After losing the case due to von Lichtenfels' connections, Paracelsus openly attacked the judges and magistrates of Basel in a series of broadsheets and pamphlets. A warrant was shortly after issued for his arrest. At the urging of a friend, he managed to escape under cover of darkness. Paracelsus was thereafter on the run.

His ambitions at Basel had come and gone with meteoric speed. In a short ten months, Paracelsus had begun and ended a courageous and innovative attempt to reform medical education in Europe. He spent the remaining fourteen years of his life writing and travelling, healing where he could, and contending with a medical profession that had closed ranks and blocked his many attempts to regain influence in the European community.

The legacy

Unlike Hippocrates or Galen, Paracelsus remained an outlaw for most of his days. He embodied the tumultuousness and vitality of an age where, for the first time, knowledge became available to those who could read. This knowledge was drawn from many new sources, and increasingly challenged the authority of both a church and a medical profession that had, for too long, held to rigid notions regarding the nature of life and the world.

Paracelsus has been lauded by some as the visionary progenitor of contemporary drug-based systems of medicine. He has also been vilified as a destructive force who subverted venerable traditions and promoted the use of poisonous minerals by many generations of European doctors. Neither view encompasses the truth that he embodied.

His main gift to Western medicine was a spirit of openness and independence that encouraged the examination and exploration of all sources of knowledge, not simply those sanctioned by the authorities and institutions that hold power at any given time. He vehemently resisted the limitations on understanding imposed by the dogmatism of humoral approaches to medicine. He viewed the body both as *integrum*, a whole phenomenon in itself, yet also sought to understand the nature of its different organ systems and their influence in health and disease. Although Paracelsus understood that medicines of all classes influenced the body in some way, he was determined to uncover the nature of those hidden substances within them that affected the body in very specific ways.

Paracelsus was equally drawn towards developing an understanding of the role of spirit and imagination in healing. Towards the end of his life, he wrote:

> If we are firm in the art of meditation, we shall be like Apostles. We shall not fear death, prison, martyrdom, pain, poverty, toil, hunger. We shall be able to drive out the Devil, heal the sick, revive the dead, move mountains. The practice of the art is based on speculation and meditation.[16]

Paracelsus represented not only a prophet of an emerging medical naturalism that would find eventual expression in a future pharmacology, but carried a deeply holistic understanding of the connectedness of body, mind and spirit.

The humoral paradigm inherited from the Graeco-Arabic tradition continued to be taught in European medical academies until the early nineteenth century. The work of Paracelsus and of the European alchemists did, however, stimulate a deepening interest in the nature of medicinally active substances and, consequently, the further development of European pharmacology and medicine. The description of elemental *forces* and *qualities* in plant medicines was soon overtaken by the quest to isolate particular *substances* that had powerful and specific effects on the various functions and activities of the body.

The grinding of glass into lenses and prisms had opened human vision to the immensity of the universe. Later, in the seventeenth century, Anton von Leeuwenhoek and Robert Hooke independently devised new instruments using lenses of ground glass, but directed their attention towards the world of living matter rather than the night sky. Their primitive microscopes showed undreamed-of worlds within a single drop of pond water. They also showed living bodies to be made up of highly differentiated cells, which were themselves composed of myriad organelles. A new vision of life and its manifestations gradually began to emerge.

Paracelsus had cast the canons of the ancients into the flames. From that time on, new technologies and new methods of analytical investigation were to drive a quest that progressively shook the venerated foundations of what had seemed to be a rock-solid tradition of medicine in Europe.

The new pharmacology

Renaissance alchemists had brought to a fine art the various methods of separating and purifying both the volatile and fixed substances within the plant, animal and mineral kingdoms. From the early 1800s, their labours began to be more systematically applied as many new compounds were separated from the more potent plant medicines that had been used for thousands of years in Europe, North Africa and the newly discovered Americas. A new generation of pharmacologists worked at extracting crystalline salts, often of remarkable power, from plants that were known to have profound effects on human physiology.

In 1806, the German chemist Serturner drew forth a beautifully refractive salt from the black and sticky exudate of lanced opium poppies. He named this salt morphine, after Morpheus, the Greek god of dreams. Within ten years, the French chemists Pelletier and Caventou had similarly drawn from Jesuit's bark, *Cinchona officinalis*, the alkaloids quinine and quinidine. From *Strychnos nux vomica*, the universally prescribed tonic medicine of nineteenth-century European medicine, they extracted the alkaloid strychnine. Within a generation, atropine had been drawn from *Atropa belladonna*, colchicine from *Colchicum autumnale*, the autumn crocus, and cocaine from *Erythroxylon coca*, the remarkable leaf that gave such powers of endurance to the tribal people of the Andes.

The discovery of chemical compounds that could profoundly alter human metabolism and experience caused a major shift in the focus of European medicine. The alchemical search for such medicines as the *lapis philosophorum* (the philosopher's stone) or *aurum potabile* (potable gold), which were reputed to cure all diseases to which humans are subject and to replenish any deficiency of *spiritus vitae* or life force, gave way to the far more modest goal of finding specific medicines that would predictably cure specific diseases. The search began for new chemical agents that would alter the natural progression of human diseases with certainty.

This search was to be dramatically realised within a short time of its envisioning, through the work of the German microbiologist Paul Ehrlich. Ehrlich was among the first of many generations of research scientists who would devote their energies to the quest for new medicines that could selectively destroy the causative agents of specific diseases. The method developed by Paul Ehrlich in his search for powerful and predictably effective medicines was to dominate the search for new drugs by scientific medicine for nearly a century.

Of drugs and perseverance

As a student in the 1880s, Paul Ehrlich had become fascinated by the microscope and what it revealed. In his doctoral thesis he investigated newly developed techniques for staining cells and micro-organisms. Through his work with histologic stains, he soon learned that certain chemicals would preferentially target particular cells and micro-organisms, and even particular organelles within cells. Ehrlich asked whether powerful chemical poisons could also target and destroy invading bacteria and other micro-organisms without damaging normal cells.

At the time that Ehrlich was asking such questions, the doctrine of specific aetiology was gaining credibility. This doctrine represented a revolutionary departure from the humoral notions of disease causation that had dominated European medical thinking for more than two thousand years. Earlier microscopic studies had established with certainty that syphilis was caused by the spirochaete *Treponema pallidum*. It was also known that a single-celled protozoan, the trypanosome, caused the devastating sleeping sickness of Central and West Africa. Ehrlich set his sights on these diseases and began looking for a drug that could kill these infectious organisms without damaging the patients who were infected.

Paul Ehrlich irrevocably changed the way in which Western medicine was to search out new drugs. His new method was disarmingly simple. It was based on a thorough and systematic testing of newly discovered chemicals on selected micro-organisms and on experimental animals infected with those organisms. Ehrlich had a superhuman capacity for perseverance in the face of repeated failure and frustration. In time, he was to become a living testimony to the saying of Isaac Newton, 'perseverance leads to miracles'.

Ehrlich tested hundreds of the new compounds that were pouring out of Europe's chemical laboratories on colonies of spirochaetes and trypanosomes. He carefully observed their effects under the microscope. A promising few were found to be capable of destroying these disease-causing organisms, but further experiments showed them to be equally fatal to the laboratory animals on which they were used. Ehrlich continued undaunted.

His efforts finally came to fruition in 1910 with the 606th compound that he tested, an organic arsenical compound. This new chemical rapidly killed both the spirochaetes that caused syphilis and the trypanosomes that caused sleeping sickness. It appeared to be well-tolerated by experimental animals, and later by humans. This compound was called *Salvarsan*, or simply 606, and proved to be the first drug in history that could decisively and predictably cure syphilis and trypanosomiasis.

Paul Ehrlich created the first 'magic bullet' of modern medicine, a compound capable of selectively targeting a specific pathogenic microorganism in humans without harming other cells, by a method that has become known as random screening. For much of the following century, the search for new drugs in Western medicine followed virtually the same trajectory as that developed by Ehrlich.

Ehrlich spent the rest of his life searching for other similarly deadly 'bullets' that could destroy the newly discovered bacteria that caused major sicknesses in so many patients. He died without realising his dream. Ehrlich's vision was not to be realised until the 1930s, when the German pharmacologist Gerhard Domagk discovered the anti-streptococcal activity of sulphanilamide.

Towards modernity

The story told here aims to identify a number of turning points in the progression of medical understanding that have had a significant effect on present developments. Although some attention has been given to the role of academic influences in the development of the form of medicine that would come to dominate the West during the twentieth century, it is important to realise that history represents a vast repository of concurrent stories.

One can, for example, trace a distinct lineage between the healing ministry of Jesus of Nazareth and the formation of early hospitals by monastic orders. Such individuals as the monk and statesman Cassiodorus in the sixth century and the nature-mystic abbess Hildegaard of Bingen in the twelfth century each held the work of healing to be more a personal vocation rather than an academically based secular profession.[17]

Healing remains as mysterious a phenomenon as it was in the days of Asklepios and the healing temples built in his name. Physicians throughout history have often managed to help their patients in ways that still remain little understood by scientific medicine.

Concepts similar to those that informed Hippocratic medicine and the medicine of pre-Renaissance Europe continue to be used with great effect by healers in traditional Chinese medicine, Indian Ayurvedic and Siddha medicine, and the Unani medicine of Islamic communities. Shamanistic practices and the techniques of spiritual healing continue to provide relief and cure for many throughout the world today.

The knowledge gained in earlier times and in other civilisations is certainly of a very different nature to that which has emerged in the West since the time of the scientific and industrial revolutions. It nonetheless continues to provide acceptable explanations of the nature of health and disease to both physicians and their patients throughout the world.

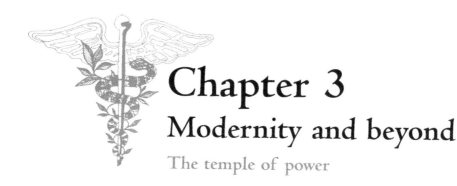

Chapter 3
Modernity and beyond
The temple of power

Medicine's position today is akin to that of state religions yesterday. It has an officially approved monopoly of the right to define health and illness and to treat illness. Furthermore, as its great prestige reflects, it is highly esteemed in the public mind. Its position is not a long-established one; in fact, it is less than a hundred years old.

Eliot Friedson, 1988[1]

Interest-based politics rather than scientific logic per se, is central to the understanding of health care in general and the relationship between orthodox and alternative medicine in particular.

Mike Saks, 2003[2]

Over the course of the eighteenth and nineteenth centuries, the factual errors of the past regarding the structure of the human body were systematically corrected through the work of university-based anatomists. Earlier notions that disease represented a punishment from God or the intervention of wrathful deities and malignant spirits were put aside as the superstitions of a more ignorant age. And the finely developed Greek interpretation of disease as an imbalance of the elemental forces and potencies that animated our being was replaced by a deepening knowledge of the nature of organic pathology and of bacteriology.

During the nineteenth century, a new generation of epidemiologists began to draw their own conclusions regarding patterns of health and disease in human communities. They soon identified the relationship between poor sanitation and disease in the squalid towns and cities swollen by promises of urban industrialisation. Sanitary engineers became bolder in their interventions, and the health of nations began to flourish as sewerage systems and piped water supplies became more freely available. With the simultaneous improvement in transport systems, urban communities began to benefit not only from the increasing availability of clean water but also a constant supply of fresh food.

A dramatic decline in infant mortality rates paralleled these developments. Scientific medicine staked its own claim as key player in this process. Developments in epidemiology, anaesthesiology, surgery and pharmacology were seen as early portents of a new and enlightened age driven by scientific knowledge and technological mastery. The earlier ways of medicine were steadily left behind as newer scientific approaches began to make their presence felt.

Many different approaches to healing were available in Europe and the New World during the eighteenth and nineteenth centuries. In the early 1800s, patients were often bled to the point of unconsciousness, and heavily dosed with mercurial purges and crude salts of metals in the 'heroic' medicine practised by university trained physicians.[3] Gentler approaches such as bone setting, herbal medicine and spiritual healing were offered by others.

A new medicine

European medicine had been irrevocably influenced by the movement of medical education into the universities during the medieval period. The new knowledge of the post-Renaissance period ignited a fury of activity in the sciences over the next three centuries. By the mid-1800s, scientific studies in anatomy, physiology, pathology and medicinal chemistry were firmly established, particularly in French and German universities. It was from these centres that the germ theory of disease and consequently much of biomedicine emerged.[4]

The character of hospitals had begun to change during the early 1800s. Rather than serving as refuges for the poor, aged and homeless, hospitals increasingly became places for medical learning and research. By mid-century, university-based medical education in Europe was firmly established in hospital environments.[5]

The situation in the frontier countries of the new world was somewhat different. The colonisation of North America began in the early 1600s. Australia received its own new settlers in the late 1700s. Like every cultural group, the native peoples of North America and Australia had each developed their own ways of dealing with sickness over many thousands of years. Although their methods were used by some among the early settlers, the methods of European-trained doctors tended to dominate, particularly in urban communities.

The first American school of medicine was formally chartered in Philadelphia in 1765. The first medical school in Australia was established a century later at Melbourne University in 1862. But until the early 1900s, most of those who ministered to the health needs of their communities in both Australia and North America had learnt their craft through apprenticeship programs or through training courses at private colleges.

Educational standards varied enormously. The curricula of the private colleges were shaped according to the inclinations of their founders and teachers. Diplomas were available to all who were prepared to attend the lectures and pay the prescribed fees. Clinical training was often rudimentary, occurring if at all through small teaching clinics. In some ways, this situation found an historical echo in many of the private colleges that offered training in the modalities of complementary medicine prior to their movement into university environments and their accreditation by government health bodies.

The character of North American medical education was to change dramatically in the first decade of the 1900s. That change was in turn to influence the style of medical education that eventually became established throughout the West.

Taking the reins

A small medical elite began to form in the United States during the middle to late 1800s. It consisted of mostly European-trained doctors, generally from wealthy families. Some members of this group turned their attention to the social and political development of their profession and became active in the newly formed American Medical Association. Within a few short decades after its formation in 1847, the AMA was transformed from a small and dispersed assembly of eclectic practitioners of low social status into a cohesive political body of great power and influence.

Others within the group directed their energies to the reform of medical education. A small number of teaching programs modelled on the European schools began to take shape in the United States. During the early 1870s, Harvard University developed a three-year medical course, and over the following decade similar programs were developed in Pennsylvania, New York and Michigan. A revolutionary new program was commenced at Johns Hopkins University in Baltimore in 1893, where all prospective students were required to have completed a college degree before starting medical studies. Those accepted into the program undertook two years of laboratory-based scientific studies followed by a further two years of hospital internship.

The Johns Hopkins model was, in subsequent decades, to redefine the nature of medical education not only in the United States, but throughout the developed world.

Of mammon and medicine

The American Civil War accelerated the opening up of a newly acquired continent. Steel mills, coal and petroleum refineries generated the materials and machinery that created a rail and road network of unprecedented magnitude within a very short time.

Economic growth was fuelled by virtually unlimited access to an expanding marketplace. Andrew Carnegie and John D. Rockefeller had drawn up the blueprint for American-style wealth creation long before Bill Gates gathered his fortunes from the silicon chip. Carnegie invested in iron manufacturing and the coalmining industries upon which the American rail system was built. Rockefeller held a virtual monopoly in US oil refining through his Standard Oil Company. Between them, they founded new dynasties of unimaginable wealth and power.

A significant part of that wealth catalysed the transformation of American medicine. Both Carnegie and Rockefeller set up a number of philanthropic trusts that made funds available to many social institutions. The profession of medicine in the United States lost no time in making use of the opportunities offered by the patrons of a new technocracy.

The AMA set up its Council on Medical Education in 1904, as early graduates began to emerge from the new schools. One of its first projects called for the systematic inspection and grading of every medical school in North America. The AMA then sought to eliminate what it considered to be inferior schools, and to support those schools that followed the scientific model established at the Johns Hopkins School of Medicine.

In 1907 the Council on Medical Education approached Henry S. Pritchett, President of the Carnegie Foundation for the Advancement of Teaching, and presented him with the findings of their first inspections. Pritchett warmed to the project and immediately contacted his friend Charles Eliot, who was at that time President of Harvard University and a fellow trustee of the Carnegie Foundation. Eliot also happened to be on the board of the Rockefeller Institute of Medical Research. Pritchett also contacted Simon Flexner, director of the Rockefeller Institute, regarding the Council's survey. Flexner suggested that his brother Abraham might be the perfect man for the job.

Under the patronage of the Carnegie Foundation, Abraham Flexner systematically visited each of the 155 medical schools in North America with a view to assessing their potential. Many doors were thrown open as school principals lined up for what they thought would be a slice of the cake. But Flexner had been well courted by both the AMA and the members of the Johns Hopkins faculty before his departure. His eventual findings were pleasing to his powerful advisers, but shocked many of the schools. In the words of medical sociologist Paul Starr:

Flexner's recommendations were straightforward. The first-class schools had to be strengthened on the model of Johns Hopkins, and a few from the middle ranks had to be raised to that high standard; the remainder, the great majority of schools, ought to be extinguished.[6]

Flexner's report helped to change American medicine from what sociologist E.R. Brown described as 'ignominy and frustrated ambition' into a profession of 'prestige, power, and considerable wealth'.[7] Paul Starr further described the character of this change:

In the nineteenth century, the medical profession was generally weak, divided, insecure in its status and income, unable to control entry into practice or to raise the standards of medical education. In the twentieth century, not only did physicians become a powerful, prestigious, and wealthy profession, but they succeeded in shaping the basic organisation and financial structure of American medicine.[8]

The AMA's first inspections in 1905 had resulted in some changes. But these were a mere shadow of what was to come after the publication of Flexner's 'Bulletin Number Four' in 1910. In the five years between the first AMA review and the publication of Flexner's report, the number of medical schools had dropped from 166 to 133. Some schools had merged and others closed down. The writing was clearly on the wall. Five years later in 1915, that number had dropped to 104 schools. By 1929, only 76 schools of medicine remained in the United States.[9]

There can be no doubt that many of the schools that closed their doors did so because of the inadequacy of their programs. Opportunism does not respect professional or educational boundaries. But the more significant consequences of this development were the loss of eclecticism and diversity within medical education, the adoption on a global scale of a singular educational curriculum, and an increasingly standardised approach to the treatment of patients.

Narrowing the field

During the decisive first decade of the twentieth century, the American Medical Association consolidated its hegemony by undertaking a massive recruitment of members. At the turn of the century, the AMA sported a membership of 8400; by 1910, its numbers had increased to a massive 70 000. This platform provided the muscle needed to call the tune in the United States thereafter.

Through the implementation of Flexner's recommendations, medical education increasingly became the privilege of the already wealthy. A short eight years after Flexner issued his report, Henry Pritchett expressed serious misgivings. He was particularly troubled by the fate of many African-American schools of medicine under the AMA's new policy, and feared the death of all medical education for African Americans if the AMA had its way. In 1918, he publicly protested the 'grave injustice done to the negro schools by the Council's de facto policy of not extending to them the same leniency given to white schools in the South'.[10]

Flexner himself was later to express disappointment at the way the AMA had imposed the Johns Hopkins model upon all wishing to enter the portals of medicine. Flexner was himself an educator, and placed a high value on diversity and flexibility in graduate education in both the arts and sciences. Paul Starr was to comment:

> Flexner . . . felt that the uniformity of medical education stifled creative work. In the years after his report was published, he became increasingly disenchanted with the rigidity of the educational standards that had become identified with his name.[11]

But by that time, the AMA had achieved its aims. Medical education in North America was now based upon laboratory science followed by hospital internship. State support had been secured for both educational programs and professional control. And competing approaches to health care were effectively emasculated and presented no further problem. The great gain had been a widespread dissemination and utilisation of scientific knowledge of disease and rational methods of treatment. The great loss was a severe eclipsing of the art of physicianship that had been slowly won over many thousands of years.

In his report, Flexner recommended that clinical positions be established on a full-time salaried basis at Johns Hopkins. Rockefeller immediately provided US$1.5 million. This was but the first small trickle of an eventual flood of funding that would be poured into the new medical education.

Over the next few years, the Rockefeller Foundation contributed an additional $8 million to set up similar full-time positions at the medical schools of Washington University, Yale and the University of Chicago. Between 1919 and 1921, Rockefeller provided a further $45 million to the General Education Board of the AMA, specifically for medical education. Philanthropic foundations eventually contributed the staggering sum of $300 million for medical education and research in North America between 1910 and the early 1930s.[12]

It should be remembered that these developments were not simply a local manifestation of political influence and financial largesse. The leverage of the immense sums of money provided by the Carnegie and Rockefeller philanthropies enabled the particular model of medicine taught at Johns Hopkins University to be universalised throughout North America. Other systems of medicine simply could not compete, and receded to the sidelines.

While these developments were gathering momentum, much of Europe was caught up in a brutal war that ravaged nations and left numerous institutions bereft. Among those were many European schools of medicine and their associated research facilities. Howard Berliner reflects:

> After 1910, scientific medicine became institutionalised as the dominant mode of medicine in the US. Similarly, in the UK and Europe, American foundations, led by the Rockefeller philanthropies, gave considerable financial assistance to the rebuilding of medical schools that had been damaged during World War I. The principle was the same as the American educational reforms, with support going primarily to research institutions devoted to the pursuit of scientific medicine.[13]

Within a short time, the new scientific medicine had come to dominate medical education and health care throughout the Western world. The hospital had become an integral element in medical education. Laboratory research had ensured the creation of strong links with both industry and new technologies. And the slow but steady discovery of patentable new drugs that could be prescribed universally for specific conditions contributed to the development of pharmaceutical industries of unprecedented magnitude.

Yet the many healing modalities that had proven their value over historic periods, and newer approaches such as osteopathy, chiropractic and homoeopathy that offered a differing perspective to that of an increasingly reductionist biomedicine, continued to be quietly practised on the margins, seemingly awaiting their own time.

Chemical factories and medicine

By the 1930s, the position of scientific medicine was unassailable. The doctrine of specific aetiology had come to dominate medical thinking, spurred on by such successes as Ehrlich's cure for syphilis and trypanosomiasis, newly developed treatments for endocrine disorders through hormone replacement, and the implementation of successful vaccination programs.

Research laboratories throughout Europe were feverishly looking for drugs that could treat bacterial infections, a source of major mortality at the time. Paul Ehrlich had set the standard with his Compound 606. Attention was still focused on the chemical dyes that appeared to be selectively taken up by certain cells. Gerhard Domagk was a pharmacologist and research director of I.G. Farben Industrie, a major German drug company that produced many of the new chemical dyestuffs that found increasing use in the textile and other industries. During the late 1920s and early 1930s, Domagk and his colleagues systematically tested the pharmacological activity of the new chemical dyes produced by I.G. Farben on streptococcal infections in mice. *Streptococcus haemolyticus* was known to be the causative agent of many common and often fatal infections in humans. Domagk had earlier experimented with a range of organo-metallic compounds, similar to those used by Ehrlich, but had found them all to be too toxic. His attention turned to *azo* dyes.

In 1932, Domagk discovered that one of the red dyes produced by his company could prevent death in mice infected with haemolytic streptococci. Although this patented compound, known as Prontosil, protected infected mice when given internally, it had no effect whatsoever on in vitro cultures of the bacterium. While pursuing these investigations, his daughter accidentally cut her finger, which became severely infected. She developed a high fever soon after and became seriously ill. Fearing for her life, Domagk injected her with several doses of Prontosil. Her condition changed dramatically. Within a few days, she had totally recovered.

Over the following three years, more than 1500 cases of severe streptococcal infection were treated by doctors in Germany with Prontosil. The results were stunning. A 1933 study reported on the dramatic cure of a 10-month-old child who was in the terminal stages of streptococcal septicaemia. But the results of these early tests were withheld from the medical community outside of Germany. News was finally released to the wider European community in 1935, a full three years after Domagk's initial discovery. Systemic streptococcal infection was, at that time, a known cause of premature death throughout the world.

The implications of the German studies of Prontosil were immediately understood in France, the United Kingdom and North America. A French researcher contacted I.G. Farben and asked for a small sample of the drug. They refused his request. The Laboratory of Therapeutic Chemistry at the Pasteur Institute similarly asked to be supplied with a small sample. They too were denied. The Pasteur Institute then tracked down the patent specifications for Prontosil, and within a short time had synthesised its own red crystals. These were then tested on infected mice. Their anti-streptococcal activity was dramatically confirmed.

It soon became apparent why the research carried out in Germany had been suppressed for three long years. The French scientists discovered that it was not Prontosil itself that killed the bacteria, but that the drug became effective only after it had been split by intracellular enzymes to produce a smaller molecule, sulphanilamide. Sulphanilamide itself had been first synthesised in 1908, and its patent had long since expired. Sulphanilamide was, in fact, one of the starting materials used in the I.G. Farben process to synthesise Prontosil.

The French soon established that the hydrochloride salt of sulphanilamide was just as potent a cure for streptococcal infection as Prontosil itself and, unlike the patented compound, also inhibited the growth of in vitro streptococcal cultures.

In withholding their findings from the world's medical community, I.G. Farben were clearly playing for time. They knew that their patent would not hold. Large and powerful drug companies are not necessarily driven exclusively by moral and humanistic concerns.[14]

Random screening and drug discovery

Sulphanilamide was discovered using the same method, random screening, as that developed by Paul Ehrlich thirty years earlier. In the ten years after Domagk's discovery of the anti-streptococcal activity of Prontosil, over 5400 derivatives of sulphanilamide were synthesised and then systematically tested for anti-bacterial activity. A handful of these have survived into the present time. British doctor and researcher Ronald Hare has observed:

> The first step that led to it [Prontosil] had been nothing more than the 'screening' of every new compound produced by the industrial empire that employed Domagk . . . . However unintellectual the method may have been, it was better than nothing, and in the end paid dividends.[15]

In a similar manner, the investigation of antibacterial activity in *Penicillium notatum* and the consequent discovery of penicillins by Howard Florey in 1939 led to the screening of many thousands of related moulds and soil bacteria in the search for new antibiotics. During the mid-1940s, medical researcher Selman Waksman tested over one thousand different species of soil moulds and bacteria. Around a hundred species of those possessed antibiotic activity, but only 5 per cent of these proved to be sufficiently non-toxic to be clinically applicable. Among them was the soil mould *Streptomyces griseus*, from which was isolated the streptomycin that revolutionised the treatment of tuberculosis at that time.

The discovery of sulphanilamide and the newer microbial antibiotics soon after were major triumphs for biomedicine. Science, technology and human determination had uncovered entire new classes of medicines of extraordinary power. By that time, the practice of emergency medicine and surgery had also become much safer and more predictable through the use of aseptic and anaesthetic procedures. The widespread successes of immunisation programs had further strengthened a growing sense that biomedicine was bringing humanity to a promised land of vibrant health and freedom from disease.

In addition, the development of steroid-based drugs derived from plants such as *Sisal* and *Dioscorea* during the 1950s enabled biomedicine to provide unprecedented control of female fertility through the use of steroid-based contraceptives, and the power to control inflammatory processes through the use of synthesised cortisone analogues. In time, such developments would enable a new wave of heroic surgeons to replace faulty hearts and kidneys without fear of the body's rejection of organs retrieved from the bodies of others.

The lengthening shadows

By the middle of the twentieth century, a reductionist philosophy built upon highly analytical knowledge of the body and of disease processes had overtaken biomedicine. Traditional sources of authority such as the Church and State progressively lost influence as science and technology became the new repositories of knowledge and power. Yet despite the numerous advances in medical understanding, and the application of a new generation of medical technologies from the 1920s onwards, a lengthening shadow began to darken the bright future promised by scientific medicine.

The reductionist approach to medicine had shifted the focus of attention largely to the body and its organ systems. The role of broader influences in the determination of health and disease was by and large disregarded. Social, economic and environmental influences on human wellbeing remained the domain of social scientists and a small group of epidemiologists. The role of mind and spirit in the creation of health and disease was simply not on the agenda. The once-human face of medicine was progressively masked by a complex mosaic of scientific knowledge, technical mastery and disease management.

Despite the cultural status, awesome technology and huge administrative empire commanded by Western biomedicine, doubts began to be raised about its actual effectiveness in delivering universal good health. It became more and more apparent that the increasingly expensive approach of biomedicine was failing to curb, let alone overcome, many chronic and age-related diseases including cancer, circulatory disease, Alzheimer's disease and, most recently, AIDS.[16]

Although the ancient scourges of leprosy, plague, diphtheria, malaria, cholera and tuberculosis had been largely overcome through quarantine, vaccination and the use of antibiotics, the effects of poverty, drought, famine and environmental degradation have in recent times seen the emergence of new and deadly viral diseases and the re-emergence of old plagues in different parts of the world. Diphtheria re-appeared in the wake of the break-up of the former Soviet Union. Parts of Africa and Latin America have similarly seen minor epidemics of cholera and yellow fever. Periodic outbreaks of the Ebola virus continue to terrorise impoverished and famine-stricken African communities.

During the mid-90s, a multi-disciplinary group from Harvard University drew attention to the widespread resurgence of infectious epidemics in a number of countries. They pointed out that the problem was not due to an insufficiency or failure of powerful drugs, but rather to changes in global ecology that have created conditions of increasing proneness of susceptible populations to major epidemics. Writing in 1995, they concluded:

> Disease cannot be understood (let alone countered) in isolation from the social, ecological, epidemiological and evolutionary context in which it emerges and spreads. Indeed, if one lesson has emerged from the spectacular failure of Western medicine to 'eradicate' certain diseases, it is that diseases cannot be reduced to a single cause nor explained within the prevailing linear scientific method: complexity is their hallmark.[17]

An increasingly holistic appreciation of the role of multiple and interdependent influences on health began to influence medical understanding. The needs of the present time call for a broader medicine than one based largely on individual biology.

Winds of change

Rene Dubos was one of the cadre of medical scientists who directed their energies to the search for cures for bacterial infections during the 1940s. Inspired by the remarkable successes of the early penicillins in war-ravaged Europe, Dubos went on to discover a number of powerful antibiotic drugs derived from soil microbes. Yet despite the triumphal mood of many of his colleagues, he cautioned against too simplistic a view of the nature of health and disease. In 1959, Dubos observed:

> By equating disease with the effect of a precise cause—microbial invader, biochemical lesion or mental stress—the doctrine of specific aetiology appeared to negate the philosophical view of health as equilibrium and to render obsolete the traditional art of medicine. Oddly enough, however, the vague and abstract concepts symbolized by the Hippocratic doctrine of harmony are now re-entering the scientific arena.[18]

Dubos' understanding is grounded in a deep awareness of the currents of medical thought that have coursed through history. Although immersed in laboratory culture, he was never seduced by the positivism of a nascent medical technocracy. His writings fully acknowledge the role of the civil and sanitary engineers of the nineteenth century who built the drains and sewers that helped remove wastes produced by burgeoning urban communities. Writing in 1979, Rene Dubos gently derided biomedicine's self-proclaimed status as a scientific discipline:

> There is more to medical science than the reductionist analysis of cellular structures and chemical mechanisms, more to medical care than proce-dures derived from the study of isolated body systems . . . The scientific medicine of our times is not yet scientific enough because it neglects, when it does not completely ignore, the multifarious environmental and emotional factors that affect the human organism in health and in disease. Reducing the normal and pathological processes of life to the phenomena of molecular biology is simply not sufficient if we are to understand the human condition in health and in disease.[19]

Dubos was as much a shaman as a scientific researcher. He understood our essential embededness within life, and the social, cultural and historical realities that condition our health and wellbeing as deeply as do physiology and biochemistry. In a reflection of the depth of his commitment and vision, he was later to co-author, with Barbara Ward, the remarkable document of a civilisation in deep trouble, *Only One Earth*.

Rene Dubos remained mindful of the power of non-rational influences in the healing practices of all cultures. He called attention to the folly of disregarding or discrediting the importance of such influences:

> Regardless of the level of cultural and economic development, all people throughout history and in the different parts of the world have practiced simultaneously two kinds of medicine. On the one hand, they have made use of drugs, surgical interventions and nutritional regimens to deal with traumatic accidents and with certain organic disorders that they could readily apprehend. On the other hand, they have developed practices of a semi-mystical or completely religious nature designed to cure physical and mental diseases by influencing the patient's mind. These non-organic healing practices—such as chants, prayers, pilgrimages, and the like—are usually regarded as irrational by outsiders, but nevertheless they often contribute to the recovery of the patient by helping him to mobilize unconsciously the innate mechanisms for spontaneous self-healing that exist in all living creatures.[20]

Dubos gave voice to that side of human nature that cannot be fully encompassed by science as it presently stands. He pointed strongly towards the subtler dimensions of mind and spirit that inform the holistic perspective.

The new ethicists

During the 1960s, British physician Maurice Pappworth raised his own concerns regarding the direction in which biomedicine was moving. He took issue with the increasingly heroic experimental procedures and diagnostic methods used in biomedicine. He cites the tragic and unnecessary blinding of eight newborn infants in a controlled clinical trial undertaken in 1954 to test a *known* relationship between the development of retrolental fibroplasia and the use of high concentrations of oxygen in premature infants. Four published reports over the previous five years had established with near certainty the relationship between high oxygen levels and blindness in premature neonates. Pappworth angrily proclaimed: 'In the name of "science", worshippers at the shrine of the controlled series rendered eight infants blind to prove what others considered to have been previously established.'[21]

Pappworth laid himself on the line when he published his concerns under the title of *Human Guinea Pigs: Experimentation on man*. He was clearly dismayed at how few of his colleagues were prepared to speak openly regarding the less desirable consequences of many of the investigations and procedures carried out at the time. His book was strongly criticised by reviewers in the *Lancet*, the *World Medical Journal* and the *British Medical Journal*. Pappworth concluded:

> No doctor is justified in placing science or the public welfare first and his obligation to his patient second. Any claim to act for the good of society should be regarded with extreme distaste and even alarm, as it may be a high-flown expression to cloak outrageous acts. A worthy end does not justify unworthy means.[22]

Maurice Pappworth was not alone in his deliberations. Across the Atlantic, anaesthesiologist and Harvard Medical School professor Henry Beecher more gently called medical researchers to attention. During the course of his own inquiries regarding the ethics of medical research, Beecher uncovered numerous examples of experimental procedures that put patients into needless danger, and in some cases resulted in their death. He originally submitted his findings to the *Journal of the American Medical Association* in 1965. The editors refused publication. He then forwarded a modified version to *The New England Journal of Medicine*, where it appeared in 1966. The article was later to be described as 'the most influential single paper ever written about experimentation involving human subjects'.[23] In it, Beecher observed:

> During ten years of study of these matters it has become apparent that thoughtlessness and carelessness, not a wilful disregard of the patient's rights, accounts for most of the cases encountered. Nonetheless, it is evident that in many of the examples presented, the investigators have risked the health or the life of their subjects.[24]

Both Pappworth and Beecher reminded their colleagues of the Hippocratic dictum first voiced by Greek physicians two and a half thousand years earlier: '*Primum non nocere*'. Firstly, do no harm. They spoke out strongly against the tendency of technological medicine to lose sight of the individual patient in its quest for greater knowledge of physiological processes and biochemical mechanisms.

Over the following decade, the authority of biomedicine came under increasing fire on several fronts. American lawyer Rick Carlson proclaimed *The End of Medicine* in 1975. Cultural and educational reformer Ivan Illich drew upon himself the collective rancour of the Western medical profession by the publication of his *Limits to Medicine* in 1976. Before the seventies were done, Australian physician and prominent member of the Doctors Reform Society, Richard Taylor made his own views clear in the content and title of his book, *Medicine Out of Control: The anatomy of a malignant technology*.

The softly spoken earlier admonishments of Rene Dubos and Henry Beecher paled in comparison to the assaults upon biomedicine launched by Carlson, Illich and Taylor. Each declared that biomedicine fell far short of its professed obligations, though in markedly different ways.

At much the same time, a number of different therapeutic approaches to those offered by the dominant biomedicine began to gain in both popularity and credibility. Increasing numbers of patients began to actively seek out the services of practitioners of what was commonly referred to as alternative or complementary medicine.

The critiques

Rick Carlson identified the disease-centred approach of biomedicine as a major problem. Significant causes of disease other than those of biological origin had been too readily overlooked. Population medicine, and social and environmental medicine, were not major elements in the biomedical paradigm. The pursuit of specialist technical diagnosis came at the cost of neglecting the broader life circumstances of patients.

> Modern medicine has only one approach to health—a wholly disease-oriented approach. Its paradigm of healing assumes that highly refined techniques and profound interventions into the body can produce health by eliminating the symptoms of disease. This has led to . . . the neglect of a blizzard of phenomena about the human being, because it does not fit the paradigm.[25]

Social reformer and former Jesuit priest Ivan Illich claimed that biomedicine had usurped the trust of patients through the often unnecessary use of technology, through its mystifying language, and through a systematic evasion of the inescapable reality of suffering and death in human experience. Within the labyrinth of technological medicine, we somehow lose sight of the essential human being. Illich also contended that biomedicine actively supports, and is itself supported by, a socioeconomic system that is inherently sickening to individuals, to societies and to the biosphere itself:

> Traditional cultures and technological civilisation start from opposite assumptions. In every traditional culture the psychotherapy, belief systems, and drugs needed to withstand most pain are built into everyday behavior and reflect the conviction that reality is harsh and death inevitable. In the twentieth century dystopia, the necessity to bear painful reality, within or without, is interpreted as a failure of the socioeconomic system, and pain is treated as an emergent contingency which must be dealt with by extraordinary interventions.[26]

Illich's critique called for the radical re-humanisation of Western medicine in order that it offer more to patients than a pharmaceutical and technological management of the pain of birth, life and death.

Across the Pacific, a newly graduated doctor from Sydney University began to express his own concerns about an increasingly technological system of medicine. Richard Taylor showed his cards early in the piece. He was one of the most courageously outspoken critics of biomedicine in Australia at the time. Taylor was an active member of the Doctors Reform Society from the middle to the late 1970s, and later gave more enduring form to his critique in the publication of *Medicine Out of Control*. Taylor cut deeply to reveal what he believes are the fear-based mechanisms of control and compliance used by some within the medical establishment to create docile patients dependent upon regular check-ups, expensive tests and questionable screening programs:

> Rather than adopt measures that can be understood and carried out by the normal average person, the medical establishment has elected to usurp

the capacity of the individual to look after his or her own health. Instead of encouraging self-sufficiency, independence and self-reliance in health and illness, doctors have persistently contrived to produce dependent hypochondriacs. Rather than emphasising change in lifestyle and mores by education and through environmental, social and economic channels as a means of tackling the main diseases of modern man, they have concentrated on doctor-patient contact and 'treatment' as the main means of prevention.[27]

At the time that it was published, Taylor's work reflected a growing disaffection with biomedicine. He called attention to the role of vested interests in medicine, to the inadequacies of the medical paradigm and to widespread therapeutic failure as he saw it, particularly in the so-called diseases of civilisation. He further suggested that pharmaceutical and technological fixes tended to mask a deep neglect of the role of social, environmental, economic and lifestyle issues in disease creation and perpetuation:

We must recognize that it is the way we live, eat, smoke (or not smoke), work, drive, exercise (or not exercise), that are the main determinants of our health. And that these actions are determined as much, or more, by concrete circumstantial factors relating to social and economic organization as they are by individual 'choice'.[28]

In the years since the publication of Taylor's book, things may have changed a little. Tobacco companies now begin to reel under an onslaught of lawsuits from many whose lives have been scorched by addiction to tobacco. Government funded health promotion bodies now encourage people to get off their couches and onto their feet. Organically grown vegetables and meats are more easily obtainable by those who can afford them. Yet fast food outlets continue to thrive, and children's programs on television continue to sport advertisements for sugar-laden snack bars and cheap hamburgers.

American sociologist John Ehrenreich went on to make his own observations. He disputed the suggestion that biomedicine actively conspires to create a state of dependency in patients, and suggested rather that widespread dependency is a cultural reality in Western, and particularly US, society. This dependency is promoted and conveniently exploited by vested interests within the medical establishment:

The dependency and passivity characteristic of modern medical care are sought by patients as well as imposed by doctors; they reflect not only the interests of the doctors and of giant corporations, but also the needs of patients. Medicine as practiced in the US may reinforce dependence and passivity in the face of bourgeois domination; it does not, however, create them.[29]

Despite the differing academic and occupational allegiances of Carlson, Illich, Taylor and Ehrenreich, there is a surprising level of agreement in their essential criticisms. All identify the presence of such factors as reductionism in medicine, medicalisation of the life process, disencouragement of independence, self-reliance and autonomy in patients, and the runaway costs of technomedicine as portents of an unsustainable system adrift from its historical mission.

Interestingly, none of these authors attributed any great significance to the increasing presence of alternative and complementary approaches to medicine as either a counterbalance or a potential restorative for the problems in biomedicine. Rick Carlson glancingly suggested, however, that more naturalistic approaches in fact represent authentic forms of healing that more often satisfy real rather than created needs in patients:

> The natural healer, whether physician or shaman, fosters and builds upon the confidence and belief of his patients. This is a crucial difference. Today's physicians create a climate of uncertainty and dependence and are consequently left with only the tools of massive intervention to effect a cure. Patients' complicity is seldom encouraged. Thus the most fundamental factor in healing is denied.[30]

These critiques gave voice to a gathering disaffection with a profession that had, over the course of the twentieth century, gained immense scientific, institutional and economic credibility, yet appeared to have strangely lost touch with its own humanity. These critiques were part of a growing realisation that medical responsibility included not only attending to the alleviation of sickness and disease in individual patients, but also the active creation of a reflective, informed and autonomous culture capable of responding healthily to the myriad abuses of persons, peoples and planet to which we are daily witness.

The rebound

The wave of criticism directed towards biomedicine during the 1970s was paralleled by a steady growth in popularity and patronage of practitioners of complementary medicine. This was met with considerable hostility from a biomedical profession whose authority was not so much being directly challenged by the work of individual practitioners, but more by the simple reality on the ground. Increasing numbers of patients were choosing to go elsewhere.

By the middle to late 1980s, the medical profession throughout the English-speaking world was expressing its displeasure through the pages of its learned journals. Sociologist Mike Saks reported regarding the situation in the United Kingdom at the time:

> The ongoing adversarial climate between orthodox and alternative medicine was most apparent, though, in the report of the British Medical Association on alternative therapy. Much of the first half of the report was devoted to documenting the triumphant march of progress of orthodox biomedicine, in classic modernist fashion. In the remainder, alternative therapies were attacked for being 'unscientific', not least because of their link to medieval superstition and witchcraft.[31]

Elements within complementary medicine that were perceived as being extreme were selectively targeted in such criticisms that were nonetheless directed towards non-biomedical approaches generally. Shortly after the BMA attack on complementary medicine, the work of the founder of the first cancer support groups based on holistic principles in Australia came under direct fire. After having successfully overcome osteosarcoma through the use of both biomedical and unorthodox methods of cancer treatment, Ian Gawler reported his experiences using dietary modification, meditation and visualisation, and natural medicine supplements in *You Can Conquer Cancer*, published in 1984.[32]

Gawler succeeded in inflaming the passions of the Australian medical fraternity. His work was ferociously denounced in an editorial written for the December 1989 edition of the *Medical Journal of Australia* by UK oncologist Michael Baum. Referring to a highly critical review of Gawler's book by Australian cancer specialist Raymond Lowenthal that appeared in the same edition of the *MJA*, Baum commented:

> The current controversy about alternative medicine in Australia as illustrated within this issue of the Journal is not some local problem or phenomenon of contemporary life, but another symptom of the virus of irrationalism that is a serious threat to the health and welfare of all nations . . . How many cancer sufferers will be denied the proved benefits of modern oncological practice while awaiting the miraculous cure that has been claimed by Ian Gawler?[33]

Michael Baum took very seriously the threat posed to biomedicine by the more holistic approaches to treatment of chronic conditions, including cancer, that were gaining increasing attention throughout the West. Yet in coming years, many of his own colleagues would begin to reconsider the potential value of other approaches, without dismissing them in their entirety.

It should be asked whether the criterion of rationality had perhaps overly determined Baum's judgements. As will be discussed in later chapters, there are principles other than those underlying rationality that determine our wellbeing. In addition, one wonders whether Baum's criticism of Gawler's ideas represents more a knee-jerk reaction than a careful consideration of the notions presented. Anyone familiar with Gawler's writings and activities will realise that nowhere does he claim to have discovered a miraculous cure for cancer. Rather, Gawler's essential message is that great personal commitment and much hard work are needed in the uncertain task of reclaiming health after a diagnosis of cancer.

The dilemma uncovered

We are presently witnessing a significant reorientation of a profession that has for much of the twentieth century focused on the technical aspects of physicianship to the detriment of its more humanistic role. Writing in the late 1970s, physician and medical philosopher Edmund Pellegrino identified the tension between the technological orientation of biomedicine and its humanistic obligations:

> Much of the discontent with medicine today arises from the disjunction patients feel between the doctor's technical role and the hieratic role which he formerly performed. We shall have to accept as a fact (an unpalatable fact, for many) that the ideal of reuniting these two radically different functions may become impossible.[34]

It must be asked whether Edmund Pellegrino has perhaps too readily accepted that the supposed dissonance between the traditionally hieratic role of the doctor and the present technical capabilities of biomedicine are unbridgeable. The immense amount of information to be acquired by students of medicine and the constant pressure of hospital internship have certainly contributed to a narrowing of the horizons of many practitioners of biomedicine. But a more fruitful approach to resolving the tension between the role of science and the role of art in medicine may lie more in the re-humanising of medical education than in a further division of labour. Such issues hinge on the simple perception of possibilities. Pellegrino continues:

> Is it more mature to assign medicine a limited role in our lives, so that we do not look for more than it can offer? Its domain could be limited to those disorders susceptible to specific therapy. On this view, the hieratic,

> personal and supportive functions could be assigned to people outside the medical profession altogether—to the patient himself, his family, friends, or a new set of therapists whose training would not be technical.[35]

One again wonders whether a clear delineation of therapeutic roles has perhaps been too readily accepted. We are here presented with a restatement of the perennial dilemma of physicianship: the task of bridging between the scientist and the artist, the thinker and the doer, the technician and the empath.

The doctrine of specific aetiology has given rise to the immensely powerful specific therapies of biomedicine. But there has always been more to physicianship than the treatment of specific diagnosable conditions. Remaining a source of hope and healing for those patients whose conditions do not respond to conventional 'proven' treatments may require a broadening of perspective rather than a limitation of responsibility. The holistic methods offered by practitioners of complementary medicine will prove to be valuable allies in this task.

The new holists

Despite strong reactions in certain quarters, the boundaries of acceptable medicine began to noticeably broaden during the 1980s. The limitations of reductionist forms of treatment were increasingly acknowledged by a vocal group of doctors who took their insights directly to the public, as well as to their colleagues.

A new wave of medical authors spilled onto the scene. American physician Larry Dossey called upon his colleagues to take on board the insights of the new physics in order to move beyond the crippling reductionism into which it was locked.[36] He has more recently totally broken ranks in writings that explore the influence of such activities as prayer on the healing process.[37]

Bernie Siegal called upon biomedicine to shed its distancing armour of professionalism and to re-awaken its capacity for human love and wonder in his book *Love, Medicine and Miracles*, published in 1986. And in the early 1990s, American researcher and physician Kenneth Pelletier urged that biomedicine reconsider its primarily disease-oriented approach, and called for a re-awakening of interest in the study of health and of those human qualities that nurture and sustain positive health through all of one's life.[38]

Putting aside the formal epistemologies that had over the previous century deemed the acceptable limits of medical truth, all possibilities were not only permitted but were actively welcomed in the name of holism, mind-body medicine and a 'new paradigm' of health and healing.

Anecdotal case histories that revealed unusual and unexpected cures were presented by those within the new vanguard of a regenerating medicine. The hidden shaman within each doctor was encouraged to emerge. The healing powers of meditation and visualisation were declared accessible to all who would give of their time and attention. The previously discounted and devalued therapies of complementary medicine were increasingly welcomed as the new physics legitimised a broadened view of the universe, where mind, matter and energy coalesced into an interdependent and interchangeable unity. It was as though the formality and measure that had characterised the biomedical approach over many decades were loosening in the growing interest in other approaches to healing that were based upon notions foreign to those of scientific medicine.

Holistic medicine represents a conscious re-acquisition of many of the principles that have informed the practice of medicine at all times and in all cultures. Hippocratic medicine was conscious of the effects of the environment and of one's way of life upon health and disease. Eastern systems of medicine similarly view the person as being in dynamic and constant interaction with environmental influences.

The obstinate Cartesian dualism that separates bodily mechanism from mental process is presently being revisited as such new disciplines as psychoneuroimmunology begin to gain in credibility and influence. Like holism itself, the role of the mind in the creation of both disease and health has been long recognised in medical culture. Paracelsus understood it to be integral to healing:

> The great world is only a product of the imagination of the universal mind, and man is a little world of its own that imagines and creates by the power of imagination. If man's imagination is strong enough to penetrate into every corner of his interior world, it will be able to create things in those corners, and whatever man thinks will take form in his soul.[39]

These more recent developments point towards a re-evaluation of much that has been dismissed or disregarded in the dominant model of scientific medicine. In the chapters that follow, the holistic perspectives embodied in the various modalities of complementary medicine will be explored in detail in order to better understand their role in the healing of the healing profession itself.

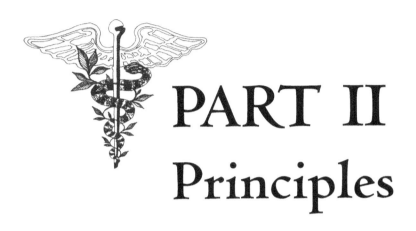

PART II
Principles

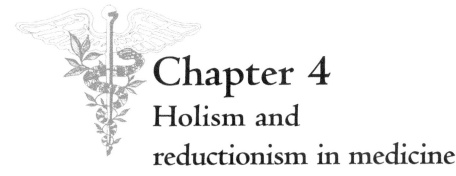

Chapter 4
Holism and reductionism in medicine
Reconciling the opposites

To a large extent, all systems of medicine except those based on modern Western science are almost exclusively based on a holistic concept integrating the body, the mind, and the total environment.

Rene Dubos, 1979[1]

Medical science has eliminated the totality of the natural biological rules in the human body, mostly by dividing research and practice into many specialties. Doing intensive, masterly specialized work, it was forgotten that every part is still only a piece of the entire body.

Max Gerson, 1958[2]

Most cultures throughout history have viewed the body as a unified phenomenon animated by mysterious life-giving forces. Egyptian doctors likened the body to a great land. As their own land was nourished and fed by rivers and irrigation channels, the human body was similarly nourished by its own flowing streams. The gods that sustained or destroyed the harvest could also bless or curse the health of individuals and nations. Egyptian doctors had power over both gods and men.

Greek doctors viewed the body as a dynamic expression of the elemental forces that coursed through all of creation. When these were in balance, harmony and order prevailed. A disturbance of that balance could manifest as bodily disease. The task of the physician was to identify the nature of any disharmony, and to activate corrective and restorative changes.

Doctors in medieval Europe continued to view the body in similar terms to those first described by their Greek forebears. But in the intervening centuries, the body had also become the great battlefield of the soul. The sins of both individuals and nations could erupt in episodes of sickness and epidemics of plague. Those sins were purged by the most powerful of cathartics and by painful and severe bloodlettings.

Every system of medicine carries an inner consistency. Each offers an identifiable paradigm or philosophy that informs the beliefs, epistemologies and methods of treatment used by its adherents. This is seen as strongly in such systems as traditional Chinese medicine and Ayurveda as in the more recently emergent forms of biomedicine, homoeopathy and osteopathy. Although each system of medicine may be grounded in radically different philosophies, they each carry an inner coherence that guides and directs the work of the healer.

Contemporary biomedicine has focused its attention largely upon the material body and based its treatment methods primarily on the use of synthetically derived drugs or surgery. As such, it represents a unique, original and unprecedented manifestation of the historic will to heal.

The body divided

Less than five hundred years ago, Andreas Vesalius recorded the first reproducible images of the systematic dissection of the human body in a remarkable series of woodcuts. His *De Humani Corporis Fabrica* (On the Structure of the Human Body) was published in 1543. It became the first textbook of the new science of anatomy. Within one hundred years of its publication, newly constructed microscopes began to reveal that each body part and organ system consisted of a mosaic of undreamed-of cellular complexes. Before long, each individual cell revealed itself to further consist of strange and beautiful forms.

The body came to be seen as more intricate than the finest clockwork mechanism ever devised. And like a clockwork mechanism, it could be reduced to many individual components that could be isolated and examined. The discoveries of the early anatomists told a very different story to that told by the ancients regarding the nature of the body.

As the body and its organ systems came under closer scrutiny, it was increasingly described in mechanical and functional terms rather than in the often poetic and metaphoric language that previously informed the understanding of the men and women of medicine. The heart was no longer seen as the source of our emotions. It served as a mechanical pump that moved blood through all the tissues of the body. The liver was no longer a source of fire that could, if provoked, flare out into uncontrolled anger. It was a large and dusky organ that received blood laden with nutrients drawn from food, and produced the bitter bile that helped digestion. The eyes were no longer the windows of the soul, but became part of a complex visual mechanism that enabled images of the outside world to be transmitted to the brain.

The new medicine increasingly severed its connections with the past. The four elements of fire, earth, air and water described by Empedocles were nowhere to be found under the microscope, nor was the human soul that had engaged the attention of both Greek philosophers and Christian theologians over the centuries. The new methods of science had unexpectedly opened the portals of medicine into fascinating and uncharted territories.

By the end of the nineteenth century, both art and philosophy had been largely put aside as scientific method was made to work in the service of an emergent biomedicine. A new generation of doctors and medical investigators began to gain in confidence. As Western medicine probed further into physiology and biochemistry, the significance of social, environmental and psychological realities on human life and health steadily receded into the background.

British epidemiologist Thomas McKeown recently called attention to some of the less desirable consequences of such developments.

> The approach to biology and medicine established in the seventeenth century was an engineering one based on a physical model . . . Physics, chemistry, and biology are considered to be the sciences basic to medicine; medical education begins with study of the structure and function of the body, continues with examination of disease processes and ends with clinical instruction on selected sick people. Medical service is dominated by the image of the acute hospital where the technological resources are concentrated, and much less attention given to environmental and behavioral determinants of disease, or to the needs of sick people who are not thought to provide scope for investigation or therapy.[3]

As one who has carefully studied patterns of health and sickness in Western societies, McKeown understands well the vast constellation of influences that can contribute to or undermine human wellbeing. He points to the limitations of a system of medicine that is based upon highly interventionist principles and a predominantly materialist view of the body. Even today, scientific medicine has difficulty in dealing with conditions that elude specific diagnosis. There are also limits to its usefulness in the treatment of conditions that are the consequence of ageing and wear and tear, or conditions for which there are no known medications.

Many have begun to ask whether there may be more encompassing perspectives from which to view health and sickness. Although new knowledge gained through the sciences of anatomy, biochemistry and pathophysiology has created medicines and treatments of unprecedented power, the role of the mind and the emotions, environmental circumstances, social and economic pressures, spiritual realities and even cosmic cycles continue to remain active in human experience.

The body in context

Eastern systems of medicine have, by and large, retained many of the pre-scientific notions that informed the understanding of physicians in earlier times. In both traditional Chinese medicine and Ayurvedic medicine, diagnoses are based more on a sensitive reading of the pulse of the radial artery at a number of prescribed points, and an assessment of such features as the patient's appearance and posture, than on blood tests or high-tech visualisations of the interior of the body.

The treatment methods of traditional Chinese medicine presuppose the existence of a series of conduits or meridians through which energies circulate within the body. Ayurvedic medicine similarly describes energetic centres and conduits within the body. These energies are said to be in constant interaction with external or environmental energies. In both systems, herbal medicines are administered not according to the nature of their active constituents, but according to the preponderance of such qualities as heat, cold, damp or dryness. Treatments may involve insertion of fine stainless steel needles into the body, the prescription of dietary changes and physical activity, or the use of breathing exercises. The overall therapeutic purpose is to harmonise and rebalance the body's energies and their associated functions.

A teacher and practitioner of traditional Chinese medicine offers the following reflection:

> The biomedical model as we know it in the West has been based on the Cartesian, the mechanistic approach to understanding, which by its very nature required a smaller and smaller look at things, and a look at things in isolation. This was based on a scientific model that felt that if you looked small enough you'd eventually find the building blocks of the universe and then you'd understand how everything worked. So therefore in looking small, the big picture—the relationships between phenomena, the holistic nature of the universe—was omitted, let's say not recognised.

This practitioner reminds us that the new knowledge uncovered by the analytical methods of science is often a partial knowledge, a knowledge that is divided from the relationships between phenomena and the contexts within which they are embedded. The methods of science have generated highly detailed knowledge of the nature of the physical body, but have failed to provide an understanding of the body as a whole, and the influence of the subtle fields within which bodies interact.

The conception of the human body in machine-like terms was first formally described by the French mathematician and philosopher René Descartes in the seventeenth century. British psychologist Helen Graham offers the following reflection of his influence upon the mind of medicine in recent centuries:

> Descartes' world-view was ... mechanistic and materialistic but also analytic and reductionist in so far that he viewed complex wholes as understandable in terms of their constituent parts. He extended this mechanistic model to living organisms, likening animals to clocks composed of wheels, cogs and springs, and he later extended this analogy to man. He wrote: 'I wish you to consider finally that all the functions which I attribute to this machine ... occur naturally ... solely by the disposition of its organs not less than the movements of a clock.' To Descartes, the human body was a machine, part of a perfect cosmic machine, governed in principle at least by mathematical laws, and this view of the body as a mindless machine has governed Western medicine ever since. [4]

The methodical analysis of phenomena and the measurement of their qualities has yielded remarkable results in the physical sciences. The acceptance of a machine-like conception of the universe led to unprecedented powers of control and predictability and new levels of understanding of the natural world. The force held in a wound spring could be gradually released through a series of gears and levers in such a way that the passage of time was marked in precise intervals. The precessionary movements of planets that had previously mystified generations of astronomers were now understood to be a necessary consequence of an earth-based perspective in a heliocentric planetary system.

The human body that had earlier been viewed as a unified organism infused and governed by elemental forces similarly came to be perceived as a complex machine of intriguing detail. Unravelling those details held the promise of new knowledge and new powers of intervention. The realisation of that knowledge changed the character of the profession of medicine in the Western world thereafter.

Although reductionist approaches have conferred extraordinary levels of knowledge and understanding of the structure and functions of the various organ systems of the body, they have been of limited value in developing a similar knowledge and understanding of the influence of mental states, social relationships, environmental and economic conditions, and natural cycles on our state of health.

The body as whole

Scientific method has determined the game plan of what is deemed good medicine throughout most of the Western world. Yet despite this, there occurred a remarkable surge in the popularity of complementary medicine during the closing decades of the twentieth century.

Such modalities as Western herbal medicine and traditional Chinese medicine were practised in their respective cultures long before the scientific revolution of the seventeenth century. More recently developed modalities such as naturopathy and homoeopathy are based on principles that differ from those that underlie biomedicine. While biomedicine rests strongly on the foundations of rationalism and reductionism, the modalities of complementary medicine tend more towards empiricism and holism.

Many within Western society are choosing to bypass the culturally sanctioned and proven methods of scientific medicine in favour of more holistic approaches. This may reflect a general sense that pharmaceutical solutions to the management of health problems are not the only way to deal with sickness and disease. It may also reflect a growing awareness that the way in which we live our lives can influence both our proneness to ill-health, and our ability to recover from such episodes when they do arise. Such considerations may resonate at deeper levels of the patient than reassurances that a pharmaceutical prescription is all that is required.

Practitioners of complementary medicine have far greater therapeutic freedoms than those of biomedicine. Each modality tends to have its own particular methods of diagnosis and treatment. Homoeopathic medicines, for example, may be selected according to such indicators as whether a patient feels hot or cold, or the time of day or night when symptoms are aggravated or relieved. Rather than aiming for rapid symptomatic relief through specific treatment, these approaches tend to focus more upon ways in which the health of patients can be directly or indirectly strengthened. This therapeutic slant is one of the characteristic differences between reductionist and holistic approaches to medicine. A teacher and practitioner of Western herbal medicine elaborates on how such approaches may be expressed in the clinical situation:

> If they came to a natural therapist or a herbalist for example, we would assess the situation, look at other factors, what else is happening in that person's body, then look at dietary factors and non-pharmacological factors to assist in the relief of the flu. We would prescribe a medicine that

will not only dry up the sinuses or whatever, but perhaps work on the liver for its detoxifying properties, work on the general immunity, boost the immunity. Perhaps maybe some digestive medicine [is also prescribed] if in the assessment of the practitioner that's at play. So yes, I would say that is the difference. And they call this the holistic approach.

This quote offers some insight into how sensitivity to bodily holism finds expression in herbal medicine practice. A patient suffering from the flu is viewed as an integrated embodiment of inter-related activities, and not simply as the walking carrier of an infection for which there may or may not be a specific medicine. The patient's presenting symptoms do not represent the total field—other factors are at work. The presenting symptoms are to be dealt with as far as possible using appropriate medication, but the deeper task of the healer includes reflection upon how the patient's own protective systems can be better activated.

In the context of osteopathic medicine, the body is similarly viewed as an integrated totality, although it is understood more in mechanical rather than organic terms. The founder of osteopathy, Andrew Taylor Still, often described the body as a machine or engine. But he also accepted that the body was infused with spiritual and energetic principles:

As an electrician controls electric currents, so an osteopath controls life currents and revives suspended forces . . . Study to understand bones, muscles, ligaments, nerves, blood supply, and everything pertaining to the human engine, and if your work be well done, you will have it under perfect control.[5]

Osteopathic medicine is based on a deep study of anatomy and depends in its evolved practice on a detailed knowledge of the mechanical workings of the supportive structures of the body. Yet, like Eastern systems of medicine, osteopathy views the body as an *integrum* and in its treatments seeks to restore the balance of the dynamic activity that underlies its workings. It was, perhaps, to this possibility that Rick Carlson was alluding when he commented:

It is one thing to treat the patient as a machine, ignoring a rich store of information that is related to health and functioning, and yet another to further subdivide the machine into its constituent parts. In the former medicine, at least the possibility existed for holistic treatment. In today's medicine, the task is nearly impossible.[6]

The holistic approach encompassed in many of the modalities of complementary medicine aims at more than symptomatic treatment. It offers an opportunity to call upon all the resources available to both the healer and patient in the task of restoring the patient as a whole to an optimal state of health.

The new holism

Holism operates at a number of levels. The individual cell is a finely balanced system in constant interaction with its surroundings. The human body is similarly endowed and responds as a totality to both interior and exterior changes. Our embodied nature also participates intimately in both mental and spiritual dimensions in ways that are poorly understood. Beyond the body, we are part of relational networks, beginning with the family and extending on to our various workplace, social and cultural groupings. Furthermore, each of us are subject to environmental influences related directly to our home and work spaces, and indirectly to the quality of the air that we breathe, the water and fluids we drink, and the foods we consume. Our overall health can be influenced at any or all of these levels.

When the body is overrun by infection, its health can be restored by both antibiotics that destroy the invading micro-organisms and by immunomodulating herbs such as *Echinacea* or *Astragalus* that increase the number of white blood cells. If, however, a patient fails to recover fully or continues to suffer from recurrent infections, it may be necessary to learn more about their familial, social and environmental circumstances in order to better understand the role of possible hidden influences and to develop more effective therapeutic strategies.

The growing literature on psychoneuroimmunology reaffirms the ancient insight that body and mind are an integral phenomenon. Our thoughts, emotions and imagination can project into the experience of our body in unexpected ways. To describe the nature of the mind is a task better left to philosophers and mystics, but we now know with certainty that the human immune system can be assisted in its activities by far more than just antibiotic drugs or herbal extracts.

There are no prescribed formulae or procedures that are universally applicable when one begins to explore holistically the various contexts within which patients live. Each situation will call for its own particular response. Canadian microbiologist Marc Renaud adds further light:

> Contemporary medical knowledge is rooted in the paradigm of 'specific aetiology' of diseases, that is, diseases are assumed to have a specific cause to be analysed in the body's cellular and biochemical systems. This paradigm gave support to the idea of specific therapies, from which arose the essentially curative orientation of current medical technologies

towards specific illnesses rather than the sick person as a whole, and the belief that people can be made healthy by means of technical fixes, i.e. the engineering approach . . .

Because of the dominance of this paradigm, the idea was lost that diseases may be caused by a vast array of interlinked factors tied to the environment, or, in other words, that diseases may be individually experienced problems of adaptation.[7]

The new holism reaffirms the universal notion that we are embedded beings and are influenced by 'a vast array of interlinked factors' that determine our state of health and our proneness to disease. A willingness to tease out the influence of these other factors represents the essence of the holistic mindset. A teacher of naturopathic medicine speaks of her own approach:

The basic philosophy of medicine I suppose is that you can isolate a causative agent and wipe that out. Which is just not our philosophy at all. We're into this labyrinth of causative processes, this causal chain of events that happen in people's lives.

Far from looking exclusively for simple solutions, this naturopath perceives a 'labyrinth of causative processes' that may underlie the creation and maintenance of states of sickness. She is fully prepared to enter that labyrinth in order to gain deeper insight into the other factors that may be active in the lives of her patients and that may be influencing their health. Although simple solutions may deal adequately with troublesome symptoms in the short term, the hidden complexities that colour our lives may also need to be given attention.

The broader contexts of health and sickness

An osteopath takes up the issue of how he feels reductionist philosophies have diverted biomedicine from the broader determinants of health and sickness:

What you have in orthodox medicine—that's beginning to fray a bit at the edges now—is the idea of disease as a sort of mechanical entity that has always concrete measurements to be found in changes in body systems and structures and processes, that are identifiably the same in everybody. The idea of specificity which took medicine a long way in terms of microbiology, in terms of organic pathology, that idea of specificity leads to an ignorance about the human soup of emotions and social interactions and ecological balances and so on that are the matrix in which illness and health arise.

In its efforts to secure control over disease processes through the tested and proven methods of drug-based treatments during the twentieth century, the Western medical community seemingly lost sight of the broader dimensions of healing. This was perhaps an understandable response in view of the immense difficulties of the task.

There is an unspoken suggestion, both within the medical community and the general population, that given enough time and money, scientific medicine will discover new drugs for the treatment of diseases for which there is at present no known cure. Such an approach is based upon the experiences of the past, where specific drugs were successfully used to cure specific conditions previously refractory to treatment. This certainly was the case with the development of antibiotics to treat bacterial infections, and hormone analogues to treat endocrine disorders. But the problematic consequences of attempting to balance increasing numbers of prescription drugs in patients suffering from multiple conditions or diseases points to the essential limitations of the project. The successful treatment of Alzheimer's disease may rest more with preventative measures undertaken during one's middle years than in the hoped-for discovery of a new drug.

It is far easier to deal with the body and its symptoms than to even begin to explore the mental and emotional lives of patients, the quality of their family, social and workplace relationships, their exposure to noxious environmental or psychological influences, or the pattern of their cycles of rest and activity. Apart from the fact that such considerations could not be easily addressed in the context of a busy practice based on short individual consultations, most doctors trained in Western medicine have had little opportunity to explore such issues during the course of their education.

Nor can it be assumed that such considerations are universally built into the undergraduate training of practitioners of complementary medicine. But holistic perspectives tend to be part of the background philosophies of most modalities of complementary medicine, and at least offer an early invitation to engage with patients at a deeper level.

A respondent who spent a number of years as a nurse in the public hospital system before training in naturopathy and osteopathy offers a provocative reflection:

The curriculum that they've got has been dominated by old school surgeons and pharmacists and reductionists. Too many hours of contact time a week, no time for the kids [students] to develop themselves and their own hobbies and interests. We've all known medical students who have been over the top. You know, rampantly busy. They're tired when they finish their medical degree, and they go into a pretty horrendous three-year internship or residency. They're pretty bent up characters by the time they're 24 or 25 years old. And I don't think they've had a chance to develop themselves. I wonder if they can jump out of the system if the system has already hurt their ability to be sensitive.

The awesome power of biomedicine is transmitted to its initiates through a rigorous program of training that starts in the dissecting room and ends in the corridors and wards of public hospital systems around the world. The world view of biomedicine is universally reinforced in standardised curricula based on analytical science. In recent decades, however, a small number of undergraduate medical programs have begun to incorporate humanistic studies into their curricula. Such developments reflect a growing realisation of the fact that medicine is as much an art as a science, and calls for as deep a knowledge of human nature as it does of anatomy and pathophysiology.

In training programs in Western medicine, there is little room for more than a dedicated mastery of the scientific and technical knowledge deemed indispensable for the practice of biomedicine. During this process, little attention may be given to the active nurturing and development of the more humanistic sides of students' natures. In addition, such intensive training programs tend to neglect any significant discussion of the historic development of medicine. Science historian Thomas Kuhn has identified this tendency to disregard earlier conceptual systems as one of the signatory characteristics of the scientific project:

> When it repudiates a past paradigm, a scientific community simultaneously renounces, as a fit subject for professional scrutiny, most of the books and articles in which that paradigm had been embodied. Scientific education makes no equivalent for the art museum or the library of classics, and the result is a sometimes drastic distortion in the scientist's perception of his discipline's past. [8]

The repudiation of a given discipline's past history may also result in a distortion in the perception of that discipline's present role and influence. An increased exposure to cultural systems of healing outside of the dominant Western framework, and to areas of learning related to social, psychological, environmental and spiritual realities might open young doctors to the notion that biomedicine, though very powerful in particular areas of disease management and control, is but one of many modes of authentic physicianship.

The systemic neglect of the hieratic and humanistic dimensions of medicine may result in a narrowing of the longer-term philosophical orientation of many practitioners of biomedicine. Holistic consciousness implies a sensitivity to the activity of subtle influences in the world. Yet the first experiences of young doctors are gained in large public hospitals where they are constantly exposed to the effects of severe diseases, and the often shocking traumas of casualty wards. In addition, the long hours worked and the confrontation with the reality of dying patients may contribute further to a numbing of sensitivities.

The very urgency and intensity of hospital-based experiences may limit the ability and freedom of young physicians to respond to the broader issues in the lives of their patients. In this regard, American doctor Rachel Naomi Remen has commented of her own experience, 'In some ways, a medical training is like a disease. It would be years before I would fully recover from mine.'[9] Thankfully, many practitioners of biomedicine *do* survive their training and quietly rediscover the perennial art of the physician as they work within their respective communities.

The issue returns again to one of balance. Graduates of biomedicine emerge from their studies with an extraordinary mastery of the techniques of biomedical investigation, diagnosis and treatment. But their knowledge of the historical progression of medicine through different ages and cultures may be limited to a short series of barely remembered lectures in their first year at university. In addition, they often have little awareness, let alone understanding, of the nature of other ways of healing that operate according to differing paradigms to those in which they were trained.

Unless one is personally drawn towards an exploration of philosophical issues, or is strongly attracted to psychological medicine, the likelihood of coming under the influence of a guiding mentor capable of awakening holistic sensitivities while coping with the rush and press of internship in the hospital system is very thin indeed. But in their professional lives outside the hospital environment, many young doctors have begun to independently search beyond reductionist philosophies in order to fulfil their own calling to physicianship.

The distancing hostility that characterised early relations between practitioners of biomedicine and those of non-orthodox medicine has clearly softened in recent years. Medical programs throughout the West are now beginning to incorporate studies in complementary or integrative medicine as part of their undergraduate and graduate programs.[10]

The new holism reflects a near-instinctive response to the need to regain a more balanced view of the meaning of healing and the deeper dimensions of medicine.

The deeper dimensions

The holism embraced by many of the non-orthodox healing modalities appears to span a number of levels ranging from bodily holism through social and environmental holism, and extends even to a cosmic holism wherein everything interdependently originates and coheres. This approach acknowledges that sickness and disease often have multiple causes. It is also prepared to call upon multiple strategies in the work of deep healing. A further understanding here is that deep healing often results in far more than the resolution or management of presenting symptoms.

Holistic models of healing are capable of accommodating the unexpected. In activating a healing process, rather than a biochemical mechanism, forces are set into motion that may have powerful transformative effects. Even as simple a change as reorganising the kitchen cupboard so as to exclude most processed foods, and the inclusion of a greater variety of whole grains and fresh fruit and vegetables may benefit not only the digestive symptoms of a patient, but the future health and strength of her children. The suggestion that a patient undertake yoga classes or tai ch'i training in order to overcome low back pain or muscle tension may not only reduce the need for periodic chiropractic or osteopathic treatments but may draw the patient towards a deep cultural study of Indian spirituality or Taoism.

Such simple suggestions may lead to a significant revaluation of a patient's priorities that may, in turn, lead to far-ranging and beneficial changes in their way of life. A practitioner of traditional Chinese medicine reflects on some of the unexpected consequences of his treatments:

> Acupuncture appears to be able to affect people at a whole range of different levels. It's almost a connecting level between the physical, emotional, psychological and spiritual levels. And so therefore when I treat someone with acupuncture, some people experience physiological change, or what they would say [is] change in the way they feel physically, their body's working and so forth. Other people may experience shifts in emotional and psychological make-up. And other people may experience quite enlightening and illuminating spiritual change. So in other words, it seems to be able to tap people at various levels.

According to the philosophy that underlies the practice of acupuncture, each of us are embedded in natural cycles of day and night, activity and inactivity, expansion and contraction, assimilation and elimination. Our physical natures are conditioned by energies that course through the conduits of the meridian system. These energies are intimately associated with outer energies that pervade the macrocosm. Disease represents a state of disruption of, or disharmony in, this entire interactive nexus. The aim of treatment is to restore the balance of energies both within the patient and between the patient and their environment.

In essence, one's relationship with God, the Tao that sustains and interpenetrates all creation, is to be harmonised. The realisation of such impressive therapeutic aims may ultimately affect more than just the symptoms that brought the patient for treatment to begin with. Enlightenment and spiritual illumination might be included as potential, if unexpected, spin-offs of acupuncture treatment.

A practitioner of homoeopathy describes her own approach to the work of deep healing:

> When a patient comes to me, I often say to them, my idea of what you need is more than I can give you, but I think if you start with me and you do so much work and we know that it is actually working because we don't bring in a whole lot of things at the same time—you know, we don't interfere with too many variables—once that's established, then I think you need to have some herbal treatment. Then I think you need to do some yoga. You may need to go and have some chiropractic. You need to have acupuncture.

The homoeopathic world view, like that of traditional Chinese medicine, sits easily with the notion that non-material influences condition our health and wellbeing. The so-called higher potencies of homoeopathic medicine contain no detectable traces of the substance or substances from which they were derived. Yet such medicines are said to carry an energetic influence that is capable of restoring order to the supposedly disturbed energies that may be the cause or consequence of disease states.

The homoeopath quoted above describes how her own style of practise may lead to similarly transformative outcomes as those described earlier by the acupuncturist, although the means used are very different. The patient is welcomed to the possibility that the clinical encounter may become the medium of profound personal transformation. The homoeopath above accepts the limitations of her own particular discipline yet acknowledges from the start that her task is one of deep healing.

This process may reach into unexpected recesses of the patient's life and experiences. It may require the assistance of other therapeutic disciplines: herbal treatment to strengthen and tonify weakened organ systems and functions; chiropractic or osteopathic treatment to restore mobility and function at a musculoskeletal level; acupuncture treatment to restore the flow and balance of the body's vital energies; and yoga practices to place the process firmly in the hands of the patient. This clearly shows how an holistic approach will often make use of a range of therapeutic strategies in the work of healing.

A new shamanism?

The philosophy of holism requires that practitioners develop an ability to think outside the square. It similarly requires practitioners to take on a broader role than that of technical diagnostician. It requires a willingness and preparedness to enter the life-worlds of patients at close range. In some ways, the radical suggestions of both Ivan Illich and Rick Carlson raised in the previous chapter regarding the nature of biomedical professionalism finds a strong resonance in more holistic styles of practise. This in no way implies that the doctor is to become feral shaman and participate in mystical ceremonies with their patients. Illich and Carlson simply affirm that the distancing professionalism associated with scientific medicine serves to limit the degree of mutuality possible between physician and patient in the therapeutic encounter.[11]

Psychologist Helen Graham describes some of the broader therapeutic goals that are intrinsic to non-Western systems of medicine:

> The aims of the healer are to help the person towards a reordering of his world view, and the realisation that he is in process, rather than static, and part of a whole rather than an isolated entity; and to assist him in getting in touch with his being and his situation through awareness of internal and external relationships, thereby achieving balance, health and tranquility. Common to all Eastern traditions, therefore, is the notion that it is the capacity for being 'shaken up' or reordered which is the key to health.[12]

The practice of osteopathic medicine, on the surface, shares very little with traditional Eastern systems of medicine. Yet an osteopath spoke in the following terms regarding his own understanding of earlier approaches to healing:

> *Previously we could have said that we were bringing people into tune with their community or their conflicts or their extended family network or kinship or some sort of passion which they'd become knocked sideways out of. Part of the healer's job was to sort of clear out all the garbage that they had got stuck with and get them back into smooth function with their environment, social and ethnic and so on.*

The above description of the role of the healer resonates surprisingly with the methods that have come to be associated with shamanism, where patients are seen to be intimately connected with their community and its belief systems. The healer's attention extends beyond the patient's symptoms and includes the larger universe of which they are a part, their social and cultural nexus. Fritjof Capra reflects further:

> The outstanding characteristic of the shamanistic conception of illness is the belief that human beings are integral parts of an ordered system and that all illness is the consequence of some disharmony with the cosmic order . . .
>
> Whereas the focus of western scientific medicine has been on the biological mechanisms and physiological processes that produce evidence of illness, the principal concern of shamanism is the sociocultural context in which the illness occurs.[13]

Capra's comment captures the essence of the shamanic approach which, unlike Cartesian dualism, accepts that we are fully integrated within an essentially ordered universe, even though our actions or inactions may influence the balance and harmony of that integration. This philosophy of participation and interdependence is yet another signature of the holistic approach.

In many ways, the historic tensions between practitioners of biomedicine and those of non-orthodox modalities reflect a deeper cultural divide that separates the technical and the hieratic dimensions of healing. Although each of the modalities of complementary medicine may carry specific treatments for specific conditions, they generally tend towards a broader view of the task of the healer.

Biomedicine tends to focus upon strategies for overcoming or managing disease states, while the modalities of complementary medicine tend to focus more upon an active strengthening of vital reserves and of health. Health is understood to reside in more than the workings of the physical body. It also embodies the quality of one's mental and emotional reality, social and cultural interactions, and participation within the cycles of the natural and supernatural world.

Clinical freedoms

Much of the discussion in this chapter has been supported by comments from educator-practitioners of complementary medicine who clearly identify with holistic models of healing. But one needs to remain mindful of the dangers of generalisation. Individual practitioners of complementary medicine, regardless of their affiliation, are free to interpret their mission in their own way and to practise according to their own inclinations. In addition, many patients who seek out their services desire only to be freed of their symptoms in the shortest possible time without attending to possible deeper causes.

Every clinician, regardless of affiliation, has the freedom to practise, within reason, whatever they understand to be good medicine. But it is important to understand that like occupational groups generally, neither biomedicine nor complementary medicine are sacramentally immune from intellectual fundamentalism, control through vested interest and human greed.

An osteopath cautions against the wholesale championing of alternative medicine as rescuer and reformer of the perennial ideals of universal physicianship:

The simple hypothesis that alternative medicine has to do with a denial of the linear mechanistic approach to medicine fits in my own mind, but when I look at some other alternative practitioners, their mind is more full of simplistic mechanistic ideas than even the most orthodox.

And a naturopath expresses his own reservations:

What I'm concerned about is that in fact a lot of the natural therapists are now becoming worse than the doctors. There is a danger within our own realm that we just become alternative medical prescribers being more rigid, being more fundamentalist, and being perhaps in some senses, more blinkered.

Such considerations reflect the seductive power of technical models of practice, where one deals more with the presenting symptoms than with the patient as person.

The clinical approach taken by individual practitioners is influenced by a wide range of factors. There is no shortage of anecdotes about acupuncturists or chiropractors who pride themselves on the number of patients they can fit into a working day. By running two or three rooms simultaneously, as some do, it is certainly possible to treat 80 or 100 patients in a day. Such approaches say more about the nature of the practitioner and their desires than about the nature of the modalities or traditions they supposedly represent.

In addition, the increasing professionalisation of modalities such as naturopathy and herbal medicine through their incorporation into university-based education programs and state-sponsored licensing and registration systems has made them ready targets for entrepreneurial manufacturers with a good nose for a growing market. This increasing professionalisation may, in itself, tempt some practitioners to take on the mantle of their former competitors in the marketplace of community medicine. But such developments more probably reflect the reality of cultural and economic opportunism than the social and historical currents that have brought the modalities of complementary medicine to such prominence in recent times.

The cultural power of biomedicine and the status of those who practise it are self-evident. The temptation to mimic the forms and style of biomedicine in order to assume power-by-association may well have overtaken some practitioners of complementary medicine. A practitioner of traditional Chinese medicine comments:

> *In my opinion some practitioners who work in the so-called alternative medicine areas are probably even more suited to working in the biomedical area because their focus is often very much on pathology and resolving pathology. But I do think that they are an aberration in a sense, meaning they're sort of out of step with the tradition they're really working with, because from my experience working with people of different healing modalities in these so-called alternative areas, those people that I've developed great respect for and insight from were the people that worked with people, not with therapies.*

Reductionism as a way of dealing with the phenomenal world may be inherently attractive to certain individuals. There is no problem here. The philosophy of reductionism has, over the past century, enabled biomedicine to develop immensely powerful treatments that have saved many lives and eased much needless suffering. Problems arise only when the reductionist view of reality is imposed as the only acceptable view. Rightly or wrongly, the quote above identifies the modalities of complementary medicine as being part of an essentially humanist tradition. Those who practise in a mechanistic or reductionistic manner are seen as off-track, and are not reflective of the *dynamis* of the traditions they represent. Psychologist Sudhir Kakar offers further insight:

> The real line of cleavage, cutting across cultures and historical eras, seems to be between those whose ideological orientation is more toward the biomedical paradigm of illness, who strictly insist on empiricism and rational therapeutics and whose self-image is close to that of a technician, and others whose paradigm of illness is metaphysical, psychological or social, who accord a greater recognition to *arationality* in their therapeutics and who see themselves (and are seen by others) as nearer to a priest. Such a line of demarcation may indeed be an expression of an immemorial dialectic in the healing professions.[14]

The notion of arationality raised by Kakar has received scant attention in much of the discussion relating to the relative virtues of orthodox and non-orthodox medicine. The often-repeated charge of the irrationality of aspects of non-orthodox medicine reflects a tension in dialectic that perhaps misses the point that both causality and simultaneity operate within the phenomenal world, and that in certain experiences rationality itself is transcended.

Ironically, as some within biomedicine move more consciously towards an incorporation of the principles of holism in their own clinical work, others within non-orthodox medicine become more reductionist in their style of practice. The reality on the ground does not necessarily reflect the expressed ideal.

Reconciling the opposites

Adherence to reductionist philosophies or holistic philosophies in medicine is clearly not an either/or situation. Each approach carries merit. Each fulfils particular needs. The phenomenon of biomedicine represents a huge cultural experiment that has transformed the profession of medicine in the West and has created near Olympian expectations of its capabilities. The engineering approach to medicine has enabled paradigmatic leaps in the understanding of the mechanisms that reflect the workings of our physical natures. The replacement of arthritic hips by titanium implants has given new freedoms to many who were crippled by pain and immobility. The insertion of metronomic pacemakers has similarly reactivated the lives of many plagued by the breathlessness and collapse of energy associated with disturbed cardiac rhythms. These are truly extraordinary developments.

But human nature partakes of more than material physicality. We also live by hopes and disappointments, by joys and sorrows, by friendships and estrangements. The complexity of our physical natures is matched by the complexity of our mental capabilities, our emotional experiences and our existential and spiritual aspirations. The men and women of medicine throughout history have long sought to understand the nature and influence of such dimensions on our experience of the world and on our state of health.

The reawakening of the mind of medicine to such realities is driven by a gathering realisation that reductionist approaches can neither fulfil completely the calling to physicianship nor satisfy many of the deeper needs of those who seek healing. We are presently witnessing a softening of the hubris in Western medicine that has for too long sought to exclude other approaches based upon differing philosophies or differing practices.

Among other things, the rise of complementary medicine in the Western world has served as a catalyst in the further transformation of biomedicine.

The various herbal medicine traditions remain as repositories of much of the traditional wisdom that has been overlooked by scientific medicine. The Taoist underpinnings of acupuncture theory reconnect us to a world charged with energy and influence. The promotion of Therapeutic Touch within the nursing profession by Dolores Krieger has subtly challenged the materialist boundaries of biomedicine. In addition, the disciplines of osteopathy, chiropractic and naturopathic medicine have each reaffirmed the primacy of notions of innate healing, whereby the body's own healing capacities may be consciously activated.

The task ahead calls for an integration of the reductionist and holistic visions, paradoxical as that may seem. That process gathers momentum on many fronts throughout the Western world.

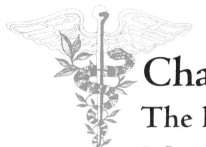

Chapter 5
The healing relationship
Reflections on the clinical encounter

The rise and fall of different healing systems ... is contingent in large part on the changing nature of the medical encounter. To understand the patterns of this relationship, one must look beyond physicians' organizations and motives which affect but do not encompass the fluid historical connection between healer and patient.

Rosemary Taylor, 1984[1]

One of the most important tools of medicine is the person of the physician himself. Medicine is concerned with the care of persons by persons, as simple as that.

Eric Cassell, 1976[2]

The Hippocratic revolution in ancient Greece saw the beginnings of a rational medicine that was to culminate in the present day as biomedicine. This revolution awakened the capacity of physicians to observe carefully and to record meticulously the manifestations of disease in their patients. It also heralded a significant change in the way physicians would relate to their patients.

The doctors of the Hippocratic era dramatically changed the methods that had been used by earlier generations of healers. They turned away from the use of the spells and charms that had been a major part of Egyptian medicine. The spoken word began to lose its power as Greek medicine turned increasingly towards the observation and evaluation of patients' symptoms.

In their desire to distance themselves from the superstitious practices of their forebears, it may be argued that these physicians also distanced themselves from their patients. They no longer engaged them in discussion, but rather, in a prescient application of formal scientific method, observed and carefully recorded the visible manifestations of disease. Eric Cassell has commented:

> Virgil called medicine 'the silent art' . . . As medicine laid aside the word, it also laid aside part of the connection between the patient and his disease and the patient and his doctor.[3]

The phenomenon of the silent doctor is not limited to the Western Hippocratic heritage. Practitioners of Eastern medicine will often make a diagnosis on the basis of such cues as gait, posture, odour and physiognomy, and through the reading of arterial pulses at pre-determined points on the patient's body. Some patients may therefore have very little verbal interaction with their physician, who quietly reads and interprets the signs, devises the treatment, and offers medication or advice.

Such styles of therapeutic interaction ostensibly enable the physician to more objectively assess the condition of the patient. They may also subtly reinforce the power aspects of a relationship where the physician represents a source of arcane knowledge that can lead to the healing of sickness and disease. Such approaches may satisfy certain psychological needs in both physician and patient. They may also further the expectation of healing on the part of the patient. But they do little to enhance an holistic evaluation of the patient and their life-world.

Hospitals and medical training

Practitioners of complementary medicine have had few opportunities to experience the reality of hospital environments at close range, except perhaps as patients or visitors. Their clinical training is more likely to have occurred in small student clinics associated with the institution through which they received their training. The early experiences of practitioners of biomedicine, on the other hand, are gained largely within hospital environments. After completing preliminary training in biomedical sciences, students of medicine in the West spend a number of years walking the wards of public hospitals.

Urban teaching hospitals are by their very nature highly structured. A medical student may spend the morning in the gastroenterology ward, the afternoon in the cardiac unit, and the early evening in a surgical recovery ward. Biomedical education also requires intensive training in the various specialities. After completing a lengthy residency in the obstetrics ward, students may then move on to the oncology or renal unit. In addition, students will often spend significant periods of time in specialist institutions such as psychiatric hospitals, geriatric hospitals or nursing facilities, and paediatric hospitals as part of their training.

Such experiences reinforce the division of labour in medicine that reflects the division of the body into its various organic and functional systems. The perception of the patient as a total experiencing individual with an inner life and an outer reality can easily be lost in the analytical maze of specialist medicine.

This situation is further reinforced in the management style that has evolved in hospital environments. Meaningful personal interaction with individual patients may be difficult to achieve in the prevailing team-based approach. Hospital patients, particularly those with multiple pathologies, often find themselves in the care of a group rather than under the care of a single physician. Medical philosopher Edmund Pellegrino reflects:

> The most delicate of the physician's responsibilities, protecting the patient's welfare, must now be fulfilled in a new and complicated context. Instead of the familiar one-to-one unique relationship, the physician finds himself coordinator of a team, sharing with others some of the most sensitive areas of patient care. The physician is still bound to see that group assessment and management are rational, safe, and personalized. He must especially guard against the dehumanization so easily and inadvertently perpetrated by a group in the name of efficiency.[4]

Pellegrino is clearly aware of the difficulty of maintaining the human face of physicianship where many individuals, each with their own area of responsibility, are involved in the testing, interpretation and decision-making processes that are often part of the determination of a diagnosis and management strategy for patients.

British doctor Michael Balint spent many years exploring the importance of the doctor–patient relationship in the healing process. Like Pellegrino, he is aware of the influence of hospital experiences in the formation of young physicians. Teaching hospitals are equipped to deal with the most severe manifestations of disease and injury. They provide a concentration of resources, skills and services for those in the community who need specialist medical attention.

Much of the training young doctors receive in hospitals occurs under specialist physicians. Although such physicians have a deep understanding of both the capabilities and limitations of their specialty areas, Balint suggests that 'they are less concerned with, and one may even suspect they do not know enough about, the total personality of the patient'.[5]

Apart from their obvious value for patients with special needs, such hospitals also enable medical undergraduates to become familiar with the full range of diseases to which we are humanly subject, and the drugs, procedures and technologies available for their treatment. Hospitals are virtual ecosystems, far removed from the day-to-day realities of community general practice. The many years spent by community physicians in such environments will inevitably carry over into their working lives and have an influence on the way they interact with their patients.

During the 1970s, Eric Cassell observed that many of his colleagues were failing to make the connection between their patients' disease and their patients' experience of the disease: 'All the doctor seems to care about are my kidneys; he doesn't care about me.'[6] Although our sicknesses may be interpreted as the necessary consequences of pathological changes in body tissues, they are nonetheless experienced by us as living persons. Our sickness encompasses not only the effects of the disease itself, but the suffering and fear generated by the symptoms, the limitations that may be imposed on our usual freedoms by the sickness, and the fracturing of our sense of self or identity.

The practice of medicine ultimately rests on the interaction of embodied beings, on persons who also inhabit social and affective dimensions. A more balanced realisation of one's role as a physician may call for the development of forms of clinical engagement that honour both the physicians' diagnostic and therapeutic skills, and the existential needs of patients. More holistic approaches invite the physician to extend their usual frame of reference.

The holistic approach deepens the therapeutic influence of the physician through enlisting the patient's own participation in the recovery process. And the holistically driven exploration of hidden aspects of the patient's reality may bring about a deepened interaction with the patient and their life-world, which in itself carries a powerful healing potential.

The physician is more than a diagnostic machine or source of therapeutic substances and procedures. The physician is the potential mediator of powerful healing forces, above and beyond any therapeutic procedure or medication that may be indicated. In order for this to be realised, however, the physician needs to know as much about the patient as about the disease.

The doctor and patient

The encounter between practitioner and patient can take many forms. It can happen in the emergency ward, with the patient in a diabetic coma, or injured and severely bleeding as a result of an industrial accident. It may occur in the office of an osteopath or chiropractor, with the patient contending with a knee injury that necessitates a complete review of their freedom to continue strenuous sporting activities. Or it can occur in a medical or naturopathic clinic with a distressed mother returning for the third time in a single winter, her child suffering from yet another ear infection. The needs and expectations of the patient will differ in each of these situations. And each situation in turn calls for a different approach by the practitioner.

Psychiatrist Thomas Szasz has given much attention to the nature of human interaction. During the 1960s, he offered a radically different interpretation of the nature of mental illness to that offered in orthodox psychiatry.[7] He suggested that much of what is considered to be mental illness in fact represents a coherent and understandable response to an untenable familial or social situation. From Szasz's perspective, much of so-called mental illness is not so much a pathological entity to be rooted out or somehow controlled, but more often represents a transitional, if disquieting, state that can, with sensitive guidance and management, resolve towards a state of greater psychological and emotional integration. In some ways, Szasz's view shares the meliorist orientation of the depth psychology of Carl Jung, who observed that mental symptoms were often reflective of a deeper movement of the patient towards individuation. The task of the therapist in such conditions is not so much to suppress or control the symptoms, but rather to guide the patient towards a state of psychological and spiritual integration.[8]

Szasz's view also anticipated a number of elements in the profoundly humanist approach to mental illness developed by Scottish psychiatrist R.D. Laing and his colleagues in the United Kingdom during the 1960s and 1970s. Building on the philosophical ideas of existentialism and phenomenology, Laing suggested that much of what is labelled madness is the inevitable consequence of the disturbed interactions and communications that often occur within families. Laing and his colleagues believed that mental symptoms were often a manifestation of existential impasse or spiritual malaise that needed sensitive guidance and support rather than medication with powerful psychotropic drugs. Laing and his group were reviled by many of their psychiatrist colleagues, and succeeded in calling upon themselves the label of 'anti-psychiatrists'.[9]

Thomas Szasz took a special interest in the various forms of encounter that can take place between doctor and patient.[10] He described three models of the doctor–patient relationship that portray the various forms of interaction that can occur in clinical environments. Szasz noted that each of the three models have parallels in more universal styles of human interaction and communication.

Szasz described his first model as one of activity–passivity, where the patient is acted upon by the doctor. This form of encounter is immediately recognisable in the practice of emergency medicine in casualty wards and operating theatres. This model also has obvious parallels in the relationship between parents and infant children. Szasz commented:

This frame of reference (in which the physician does something to the patient) underlies the application of some of the outstanding advances of modern medicine (e.g. anaesthesia and surgery, antibiotics, etc.). The physician is active; the patient passive. This orientation has originated in— and is entirely appropriate for—the treatment of emergencies . . . 'Treatment' takes place irrespective of the patient's contribution and regardless of the outcome.[11]

His second model is that of guidance–cooperation, wherein the physician, as repository of specialised medical knowledge, leads the patient through a course of treatment or medication that will cure their disease or provide relief from their symptoms. The willing cooperation of the patient is a necessary element in this interaction. In broader terms, the guidance–cooperation model shares much with the relationship between parents and adolescents. Szasz claimed that most clinical interactions in biomedicine are based on this model.

The third model is that of mutual participation between doctor and patient. This model is based more on equality between the doctor and patient than upon the power relations that characterise the first and second models. The relationship has more in common with a friendship or partnership than a formal or professional relationship. It is based on the development of a strong empathy between doctor and patient through which the doctor helps the patient to help themselves. According to Szasz, this style of relationship is favoured by patients who tend to be self-reliant and who value their personal autonomy. He further notes that working within this model is particularly helpful for those patients with chronic conditions that are generally refractory to cure by biomedicine. Szasz concluded: 'The model of mutual participation . . . is essentially foreign to biomedicine.'[12]

The ground of biomedicine has shifted noticeably in the half century since Szasz first described his threefold model. Michael Balint's work during the 1950s and 1960s did much to stimulate an interest in the importance of more empathic modes of clinical interaction. Relational styles based on mutual participation between physician and patient have become increasingly common in the intervening decades, and can no longer be described as being 'essentially foreign to biomedicine'.

The healing partnership

As will become evident, the practitioner–patient relationship that tends to occur in complementary medicine conforms more to Szasz's third model of mutual participation than to the more technically oriented or paternalistic styles implied in the first and second models. This model of interaction is central to the practise of holistic medicine. A practitioner of naturopathy views his interactions with patients in the following terms:

> It really is a partnership. I always try and make it a sense of equality there, that I am also on a journey, that I am not perfect. And I think that's an important component of establishing that relationship. It really is an equality.

The above comment reflects this particular naturopath's preferred relational mode, which is clearly based upon mutuality. The terms *partnership* and *equality* show that he assumes some degree of intellectual and intentional parity between himself and the patient; there is little distancing professionalism to interpose between himself and the patient. He also acknowledges his own fallibility and the common humanity between himself and his patient, and views the practitioner–patient relationship as a journey towards goals that may or may not be possible to realise.

This practice style mirrors the ethos of many complementary medicine practitioners whose relational modes have not been so strongly shaped by many years in hospital environments. The cultural authority that is near-universally bestowed upon practitioners of biomedicine is foreign to most practitioners of complementary medicine who, despite increasing community patronage, continue to remain on the edges of orthodoxy. In itself, this situation will tend to encourage a more informal relational style where there is less social distance between physician and patient. The practitioner can more freely disclose their own uncertainties and vulnerabilities. Eric Cassell recounts a revealing episode between himself and a young medical student:

> 'When am I going to be like that?' said one of the medical students I was teaching at the time. 'Like what?' 'Like Dr X. You know ... so sure of myself.' I think I was honest enough to say that like Dr X. the student would probably learn to appear sure of himself; but if he were really good, he would never be sure of himself.[13]

The training methods of biomedicine tend to reinforce the separation between physician and patient. As repositories of medical knowledge and participants in the rituals of birth and death, biomedical doctors inhabit a reality somewhat removed from the banality of daily life. As mediators of powerful technologies that render the body transparent and reveal the hidden sources of our sickness and distress, they wield both control and influence. Yet aside from the tests and the procedures, the clinical encounter is essentially a meeting between two persons. Consider the following comment from a practitioner of osteopathy:

Our society expects interaction. They expect to be met by their practitioner. They don't expect to be lorded over or advised to . . . I have to show myself. I can't sit behind anything. I think they are principles of natural medicine that could well and truly go into orthodox medicine—go back to orthodox medicine. Because they can do it. They're dealing with human beings so they've got to, you know.

Of all the modalities represented in complementary medicine, osteopathy would appear to be the least likely to accommodate the interactional model of equality and mutuality in the clinical relationship. The very nature of the osteopathic approach requires the practitioner to diagnose structural disturbance through careful history-taking, observation and palpation and then to provide skilled corrective treatment and preventive advice where possible. The osteopath is clearly in charge. Yet the quote above indicates a finely honed appreciation of the importance of mutuality in therapeutic encounters. Disclosure is not the sole prerogative of the patient. The physician is also to disclose himself or herself in this interaction and to meet the patient rather than simply treat the patient. There is also a suggestion here that biomedicine has somehow forgotten or perhaps abandoned an essential aspect of the healing encounter. Psychologist Howard Stein comments:

We could say that in abjuring the intimacy of the clinical relationship for that of objectivity, professionalism, control, and protective distance from patients, modern biomedical physicians considerably diminish their capacity to heal. For they can best heal who permit themselves to suffer from their patients, not they who have the demeanor of an Aristotelian unmoved mover who interposes medicine between him or herself and the patient.[14]

Interestingly, Stein does more than simply draw our attention to the formalism and distancing that can characterise the interaction between physician and patient in biomedicine. He suggests that in itself such an approach may actually diminish the healing potential of the encounter. Howard Stein also points to the crucial importance of co-presence and human empathy in the healing relationship. A practitioner of traditional Chinese medicine throws further light on this:

I don't go in assuming I am going to be looking for a micro-organism or I'm going to be looking for some sort of organic pathology. I have no idea what I'm going to be looking for. I'm not going to be looking for anything. I'm going to let that person and their experience move me to a place where they're experiencing disharmony with their life and then look with them and see what we can do together about it.

Like the naturopath quoted earlier, this practitioner also enjoys the freedom of a practice unharried by potentially life-threatening conditions or the press of an overcrowded waiting room. In such an environment, there is no longer the urgency of establishing an immediate diagnosis or identification of pathology. This comment reflects the more holistic orientation of Eastern approaches where illness is interpreted in broader terms than physical pathology. It also echoes Thomas Szasz's own description of the third model of mutual participation: 'The third category (of mutual participation) differs in that the physician does not profess to know exactly what is best for the patient. The search for this becomes the essence of the therapeutic interaction.'[15]

Our practitioner offers simple co-presence as his primary contribution to the healing encounter. Through a mutual exploration that is based more on subjective and experiential issues centring on notions of harmony and disharmony than on the objective identification of specific pathology, this practitioner mirrors a differing perspective to that of biomedicine.

Reflected in the above comment is an expression of what could be called the 'zen mind', where one puts aside all preconceptions in order to gain clarity and be fully present to the immediate situation. This form of attention is not the exclusive domain of Eastern approaches to medicine; it has been identified by Canadian medical educator Ian McWhinney as one of the signatures of evolved physicianship:

> Listening is . . . a skill, a state of mind, and a way of being a physician. Attentive listening does not mean that we are unresponsive. Without the intrusion of distracting thoughts and emotions we can respond with empathy and compassion. As clinicians, too, we heighten our awareness of the patient's symptoms. Learning to listen is not so much adding a skill as becoming a different kind of physician.[16]

The holistic practitioner is content to defer judgement, preferring to be attentively present rather than continually weighing up possibilities during the clinical engagement. There are no formulary responses to the patient's disclosures, but rather a comfortable acceptance of uncertainty and a readiness to negotiate consciously with the patient regarding the best way to deal with their experience of pain or sickness.

The art of listening

In order to discover what is best for the patient requires a shift in the practitioner's focus. Once it is established that the patient is not suffering from a life-threatening condition requiring decisive and immediate intervention, the practitioner can allow the patient to tell their story so as to obtain a broader picture. This is essential to an approach that aims to uncover the balance of influences that impinge upon health or sickness. Without an in-depth knowledge of the patient and their life-world, one cannot uncover the subtler determinants of their wellbeing. And without establishing a relationship based upon a respectful and attentive mutuality, one is unlikely to get even to first base.

A homoeopath offers some insight into how the pursuit of an holistic understanding may be expressed in the clinical context:

> I am interested in the nature of the complaint. But beyond that, I'm interested in their physical characteristics, what stamps them as an individual, what is different about them, what they particularly like and dislike with regard to their physical bodies. And also I'm very interested in their early childhood, their teenage years, the choices they've made when they left school, and how their careers developed, and how their family life is, and how their relationships with people are.

This homoeopath is both comfortable and familiar with the notion that sickness and disease can more often be determined by multiple influences than by singular specific causes. Many aspects of the patient's life are seen as relevant to the discussion. The clinical discussion will therefore range far beyond the body and its discomforts. Mental and emotional patterns, the familial and social nexus may all provide clues to the meaning of an illness episode or of lingering malaise. This quote also gives a strong sense of the detail sought and the range of experiences that may be explored in a holistically based consultation. Lifestyle and dietary patterns are central considerations, and form the nucleus around which restorative changes in the patient's life may begin to turn. Such knowledge simply cannot emerge in a short or hurried consultation. Our respondent continues:

> Look at the whole picture, spread it out. Why is this person having this problem? Ah! Because this, this and this has happened in the last three years . . . they don't do a lot of exercise. I go through the diet in detail, what they're eating, what time they get up in the morning, what time they go to work, the whole day. I like to know exactly what they do with their time so that I have an idea of where things are going astray.

Through opening up the circumstances of the patient's life-world in this manner, this homoeopath seeks to gain insight into the often unconscious patterns that can subtly undermine health. Potentially negative environmental influences and social tendencies may similarly come to light, and this will increase the likelihood of finding restorative rather than palliative solutions to the patient's problems. Such an approach clearly requires more than an encyclopedic knowledge of pathophysiology and differential diagnosis. More importantly, it requires a desire and a willingness to seek out a deep knowledge of the life-world of the patient in order to uncover the less obvious causes of disharmony or disturbance.

Michael Balint has suggested that the very style of history-taking that young doctors are trained in may limit their receptivity to or interest in the more subtle influences that often contribute to a patient's condition. Balint speaks strongly of the importance of personal sensitivity in the physician if there is to be any success in uncovering the life-world of patients:

> If the doctor asks questions in the manner of medical history-taking, he will always get answers—but hardly anything more. Before he can arrive at what we called 'deeper' diagnosis, he has to learn to listen. This listening is a much more difficult and subtle technique than that which must necessarily precede it—the technique of putting the patient at ease, enabling him to speak freely. The ability to listen is a new skill, necessitating a considerable though limited change in the doctor's personality.[17]

This comment points to a shift in the locus of control in the clinical encounter. The physician is no longer the directive authority figure or knowledgeable technician eager to secure a rapid diagnosis. Before anything else, the task of the physician is to put the patient at ease. This requires firstly a reading of the subtle clues that reveal the emotional state of the patient, whether they are relaxed or tense, whether they are expressive or guarded when they enter the consulting room. It also assumes a calm presence and steady equanimity on the part of the physician. These highly personal attributes are not necessarily everyone's birth-right, but may require active cultivation in order to become an established part of one's nature. Empathic interaction is a two-way street. While the physician becomes mindful of the emotional state of the patient, the patient is simultaneously reading the emotional state of the physician. Eric Cassell elaborates:

> Both the doctor and the sick person become exquisitely sensitive to each other. Thus the sick person is as able to sense anxiety on the part of the doctor as the doctor is on the part of the patient. Indeed, that openness of the flow of feeling back and forth enables the physician to use his own feelings in the presence of the patient for therapeutic purposes. What is required is that the physician be prepared to accept the fact that a feeling within him can come from the patient.[18]

This state of sensitivity and openness between physician and patient reflects the strong mutuality that can be established under certain conditions. Cassell also reflected: 'but to be open is to be physically and emotionally endangered'.[19] If physicians refuse to accept that state of vulnerability and remain emotionally closed to patients, they may fail both their patients and themselves.

Holistic sensitivity is not simply acquired at will. It may be that certain individuals are by nature more attuned to such approaches. The physician must be prepared to experience some vulnerability and uncertainty. Similarly, the physician needs to recognise that beyond particular methods and techniques, there remains something within human relationship that is capable of profoundly affecting the wellbeing of another.

The capacity to thoughtfully reflect in an integrative rather than analytic manner can be awakened and actively developed in students and practitioners of the healing professions. The experiences gained by health care practitioners during their early training will, in the longer term, strongly influence the methods they adopt in their lives as community physicians.

The sensitive physician

Holistic approaches enable the physician to remain useful to patients even in circumstances where the methods of biomedicine may be of limited value. This is particularly the case in the management of chronic conditions, and conditions for which there are no known biomedical treatments. To take on such tasks requires a major commitment on the part of the physician. As mentioned earlier, the relational model based upon mutuality and equality may provide the most appropriate means whereby, in such circumstances, the encounter between physician and patient can become most useful.

To work in such a manner requires a shift in the physician's centre of gravity. Rather than assuming the role of adviser or authority figure, the physician needs to now follow the patient and to be fully present to the subtle communications that pass between them. This approach represents, in some ways, an act of faith. The physician remains open to the possibility that useful insights into the patient's needs may arise during the exchange. An osteopath describes his own experience:

In our work, we work at levels of anatomical refinement and subtlety that—provided we're slow and thoughtful and allow space to feel without predicting what we are going to feel—allow feelings to emerge. We pick up huge ranges of things about people that we integrate into an intuition or realisation. And many of us rely on that sort of capacity to integrate in

*order to diagnose. And it becomes ordinary to us to pick up an awful lot
of things about people.*

Although this comment reflects the experience of an osteopath, it is
equally applicable to any clinical interaction that is based on a slow and
thoughtful approach. Such approaches assume that the physician has made
a conscious choice to take a less directive role in the clinical encounter. The
physician then becomes tuned to the delicacy and nuance of the interactions
with their patient in the quest to develop a global or holistic understanding
of their life-world. This requires an empathic sensitivity. Psychologist Rollo
May describes the process in the following terms:

> This is empathy. It is the feeling, or the thinking of one personality into
> another until some state of identification is achieved. In this identification
> real understanding between people can take place; without it, no under-
> standing is possible.[20]

A practitioner of herbal medicine elaborates:

> I think sensitivity in the practitioner–patient relationship is very important.
> I think with sensitivity the practitioner is able to tap into the needs, into an
> understanding of the patient, whereas if one is not sensitive—and I'm
> using the word abstractly here—I feel that blocks out an understanding of
> the patient.

Both osteopath and herbalist have clearly accepted that their task requires
more than a rapid diagnosis and provision of treatment for their patients.
They each seek a deeper understanding of their patients in order to more
fully realise their task. The understanding sought is of a different order to
that acquired through a reading of the results of body scans or blood tests.
Holistic understanding derives from a reflective attention to the total
presence of the patient, and to the physician's own subtle reactions and
responses to the patient. Both respondents voice in their own way the nature
of empathic attention as reflected in clinical experience. Such considerations,
however, only become meaningful when the physician can give enough time
in the clinical consultation to allow such understandings to come to light.

Time is money or time is the healer?

Holistic medicine represents more than a differing philosophy to that of
reductionist biomedicine. It calls for a near-revolutionary change in the

clinical style that has come to be associated with biomedicine. The holistic consultation is an open-ended experience. It serves a greater purpose than the relief or control of symptoms through medication. Holistic medicine accepts that we are multidimensional beings whose health resides in more than the state of our biochemistry and organ systems.

The practice of holistic medicine may be likened to an organic process that can neither be hurried nor forced. Its essential aim is transformational; both practitioner and patient are changed by the process. The practitioner acquires a deep knowledge of the patient, while patients acquire a deeper knowledge of themselves. But such knowledge cannot be gained in a standard short consultation. A practitioner of homoeopathy observes that:

> There is no way that you can start to really look at the deeper levels of what a person is doing in their diet or in their lifestyle or in their thinking within a five or ten minute consultation.

This statement points towards one of the major differences between the holistic or naturalistic consultation and the biomedical consultation—the time given to patients.

The short consultation has become one of the signatures of biomedical practice in the Western world. It appears to be one of the consequences of a way of thinking that looks for drug-based solutions to what can often be complex problems. Such solutions include the prescription of anti-inflammatory agents and analgesics for joint and muscle pain, the use of hypotensive medication for the treatment of high blood pressure, and the prescription of antidepressant or anxiolytic drugs for the treatment of troublesome mental states.

Apart from methodological and philosophical considerations, more pragmatic concerns for the economic aspects of clinic management may also contribute to the prevalence of high turnover, short-consultation styles of medical practice. An osteopath reflects:

> I wonder if they're under pressure from overheads, that's just as business people. Because the way the business system is set up in medicine, in orthodox medicine, it's quite different from the way we practice. We generally practice as sole practitioners. Some of us mix it in. We basically take our receipts and we just pay some overheads. Medical centres often are owned by entrepreneurs, or big top doctors or a radiologist. And they employ GPs and they let them take home 40 per cent of their takings.

Many newly graduated doctors enter their professional life as junior partners or take on sessional work in entrepreneurial clinics. In such situations, consultation times are determined by the appointment book, and waiting rooms are rarely empty. Apart from the high establishment cost of large clinics, there are also significant day-to-day running costs to be met. Hippocratic ideals may become an early casualty in the daunting task of balancing the books in a high turnover, entrepreneurial practice. The osteopath quoted above observed that most independent practitioners of complementary medicine tend to operate far more simply and live under fewer financial pressures. This in itself allows greater freedom to develop a more leisurely style of practice, where individual patients can be given the time necessary for the depth consultation favoured by more holistic styles. A practitioner of herbal medicine continues:

> *The orthodox medical people are limited by time restraints. I believe Medicare [allows for] only ten minutes, that's what it's geared up against. Whereas our lot, we go for about an hour in the first consultation. Generally speaking. So therefore we have a lot more interaction with the patient. I aim to understand the totality of that person, not just the presenting clinical features which are at that stage prominent in that person's situation. But there are medical doctors who are into alternative medicine, natural therapies, and I know a couple of them, they are ex-students. They actually do spend an hour with their patients. Now is there a difference between an hour they would spend and an hour which, say, I would spend? I would say, no there is not. I believe that our goals would be similar.*

Here, the same essential message is repeated: it takes time for the physician to develop a holistic understanding of the patient's situation. The holistic consultation does not revolve around the drawing out of information from the patient, or a sleuth-like analysis of subtle clues that may emerge in the discussion. The physician and patient are to enter a mutual psychic space wherein each can be simply present to the other. Insight into the hidden possible causes of the patient's symptoms can more readily arise under such circumstances. This approach has more in common with the methods of psychological medicine than with the diagnostically oriented approach of biomedicine, and is equally driven by an understanding that health and disease are as much influenced by mental and emotional realities as by physical factors.

Towards a new approach

During the 1950s, British doctor Michael Balint worked closely with a number of colleagues in both general practice and psychiatric medicine with a view to exploring the deeper potential of the doctor–patient relationship as an agent of healing in itself. Their conclusions did much to re-awaken the mind of medicine to the role of psychological factors in both the creation of disease and the activation of healing. Balint called for a re-evaluation of the more personal dimensions of physicianship. In a particularly revealing comment, he pointed to what may be a major blind spot in general community practice:

> It is generally agreed that at least one quarter to one third of the work of the general practitioner consists of psychotherapy pure and simple. Some investigators put the figure at one half, or even more, but, whatever the figure may be, the fact remains that present medical training does not properly equip the practitioner for at least a quarter of the work he has to do.[21]

The goals of which our practitioner of herbal medicine earlier spoke include not only detailing the patient's immediate circumstances, but more importantly the creation of conditions within the clinical encounter whereby the hidden details and circumstances behind a patient's illness may more readily emerge. This approach enables the physician to establish a 'deeper' diagnosis, and to negotiate possible restorative strategies with the patient. In addition, the interaction itself may carry unexpected consequences. Eric Cassell comments:

> No one knows how the physician is able to have an influence on a patient's illness apart from explicit medical or surgical treatments, but this is the process. Current research is increasingly revealing the influence of mind on immunity and other body functions, so there should be little surprise that doctors are also able to affect the patient's physiological processes. No one doubts that doctors have an influence on their patients' state of mind—we are of a piece, affecting one part alters the whole.[22]

To call such influences 'placebo effects' is to demean the powerful reality that unites physician and patient. The capacity to positively influence the state of mind of patients is potentially available to any physician who recognises the value of a holistic perspective and who is prepared to take the necessary time. An osteopath reflects further:

> It is therapy when you're giving time to someone and listening and not thinking, 'My God, I'm running forty minutes late'. If you're giving that time to them in skilful listening, wandering a little bit, starting to chat a little bit about lifestyle, those things may reveal diagnostic clues. And you're not going to get them in ten minutes. You can't be that skilled. Time is what is necessary.

This affirms the importance of simple co-presence and an attentive attitude in the open-ended clinical encounter. This osteopath also considers the act of skilful listening to be a therapy in itself. The cultivation of an unhurried mind-set on the part of the physician may invite the patient to a relaxed self-disclosure. Although direct questioning will usually elicit direct answers, what is sought by the holistically inclined physician tends to be far more elusive, and may need to be realised through the unspoken communication that constantly occurs during clinical interactions.

The methods of biomedicine are founded on a century-long refinement of knowledge and millennia of experience. The *terra incognita* of human pathophysiology has been finely charted and largely brought to subjection by the methods of surgery and pharmacology. The technical dimensions of biomedicine are now routinely mastered by all who have served their apprenticeships in the lecture rooms, post-mortem theatres and patient wards of public hospitals. A new frontier, however, has begun to open up. In reality, this frontier has always been there. Eric Cassell describes it in the following terms:

> The job of the twenty-first century is the discovery of the person—finding the sources of illness and suffering within the person, and with that knowledge developing methods for their relief, while at the same time revealing the power within the person as the nineteenth and twentieth centuries have revealed the power of the body.[23]

This frontier requires a new paradigm of exploration. The earlier revolutionary developments that brought biomedicine to such a high pitch of technical perfection were based on a deep and probing search of body tissues, the understanding of biochemical mechanisms and the harnessing of new technologies. Charting the new frontier in the healing mission will require coupling these with different skills and different methods. The explorations that lie ahead encompass the uncertain domains of relationship and empathy, of healing intention and loving presence.

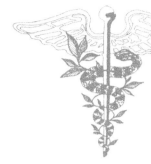

Chapter 6
The therapeutic aims of holistic medicine
Restoring the body, empowering the mind

It is assumed that the body can be regarded as a machine whose protection from disease and its effects depends primarily on internal intervention. The approach has led to indifference to the external influences and personal behavior which are the predominant determinants of health.

Thomas McKeown, 1976[1]

As individuals, we have the power and the responsibility to keep our organism in balance by observing a number of simple rules of behavior relating to sleep, food, exercise and drugs. The role of therapists and health professionals will be merely to assist us in doing so.

Fritjof Capra, 1983[2]

Over the course of the past century, Western medicine has charted the nature of disease and its manifestations to a degree that could only be dreamed of by ancient physicians. The physical and biochemical markers of most diseases have now been identified, and practitioners of biomedicine have become expert in both disease diagnosis and the determination of appropriate therapeutic interventions. But this is only part of the story. The art of medicine is based on more than a deep knowledge of the nature of disease and its treatment. It resides equally in a deep knowledge of health and the means whereby it can be maintained and furthered.

Many of us appear to live as though the gift of health can withstand all the excesses and seductions of an enlightened free-market society. From an early age, our children are entertained by television images within a stream of advertisements urging them to enjoy the delights of confectionery and big-name fast foods. We continue to be enticed in the same way throughout the course of our adult lives. There appears to be a widespread ignorance of the traditions of medicine that have long recognised the relationship between the food we eat and the state of our health.

Many people believe that modern medicine can overcome most of the diseases to which we can fall prey. If one accepts that most or all sickness can be cured by modern medicine, there is little need to actively build up our health through personal effort or careful attention to our patterns of living. Australian physician Richard Taylor has observed:

> While the majority of people believe that most diseases are curable, or at least eminently treatable by medical professionals using modern drugs and equipment, it is difficult to achieve the momentum on an individual and collective level to effect change in unhealthy habits and lifestyles. Whilst people believe that diseases are isolated, biological phenomena which are unrelated to environmental factors, real preventive medicine cannot be successful.[3]

One of the major problems confronting medicine today is precisely that of changing ways of living that are inherently damaging.

Identifying the problem

The ability of Western medicine to diagnose diseases with certainty represents one of its great gifts to the present age. Practitioners of both biomedicine and complementary medicine are in complete agreement that such diagnostic capabilities should be used for the benefit of all patients. But paths will often diverge once a diagnosis is established and therapeutic strategies are to be decided upon.

Biomedicine has, by its nature, tended to single out specific causes for given conditions and sought out specific interventions for the treatment of such conditions. This approach reflects its reductionist orientation. Holistic approaches, on the other hand, view disease symptoms as often representing the final manifestation of a complex web of causal influences, each of which contributes to the development of the symptoms.

A patient presenting with back and neck pain may be prescribed anti-inflammatory or analgesic medication. Yet a careful physical examination may reveal restrictions in spinal mobility that can be corrected by manipulative adjustments and a program of daily exercises.

A school teacher may present with smouldering symptoms including persistent coughing, sore throat, night sweats and mild headaches that have persisted through two courses of previously administered antibiotics. Blood tests may confirm the persistence of infection and another course of antibiotics may be prescribed. Yet a closer look at her circumstances will reveal a heavy workload that requires late-night and weekend corrections, and much time spent at staff meetings in the company of fellow teachers, many of whom are experiencing similar symptoms. Regaining her health may require more than soldiering on with the help of antibiotics and painkillers.

Establishing the nature of a given condition and prescribing appropriate medication is one thing. Uncovering the often hidden influences behind the development of that condition, however, may require a degree of skilful probing and thoughtful reflection on the part of the physician. This comment offered by Paracelsus nearly five hundred years ago continues to remain relevant:

> Now they say when I come to a patient, I know not immediately what ails him, but I need time to find it out. It is true . . . I desire to approach from day to day, the longer, the closer to the truth. For with hidden diseases it is not as with the recognising of colours. In colours one sees well what is black, green, blue, etc. But if there were a curtain before it, thou wouldst not know.[4]

There are often many curtains between the symptoms that reflect the presence of disease and the background causes of those symptoms.

Empowerment and the patient

The therapeutic strategies of biomedicine revolve largely around the use of powerful pharmaceutical drugs. Relatively little attention is given to the task of activating the inherent and often remarkable healing capacities present within patients themselves. Where such healing capacities become manifest through means other than the administration of a drug or specific procedure, they are commonly dismissed as non-specific or placebo effects.

The practice of biomedicine is supported by a clinical style that places the doctor squarely in charge. As has been noted in the previous chapter, there is little scope for mutuality or negotiation within such a framework. The practice of holistic medicine turns more upon a process of discussion and negotiation whereby the practitioner gains detailed knowledge of the patient and their life circumstances in order to guide them towards a deeper awareness of the nature of their condition. This represents not only a power-sharing arrangement but more importantly serves in the longer term to strengthen the patient's will to autonomy and self-reliance. A practitioner of naturopathic medicine describes his own approach:

> *We honour the symptoms that they come in with, but it can often open up completely different territory that they might never have contemplated, and that starts them literally on a journey of discovery and exploration. And in that process they also become more self-empowered which is a key word that I keep focusing on with my clients, because the medical paradigm is very much disempowering.*

This naturopath is clearly interested in more than the immediate control or elimination of symptoms. The patient's symptoms represent the point of entry beyond which a detailed review of their life and circumstances can begin. The practitioner serves as catalyst in a process that leads to deepening self-knowledge on the part of the patient. Such an approach enables both practitioner and patient to gain insight into patterns of behaviour that may be undermining the patient's health.

This form of therapeutic encounter can bring about far-reaching changes in the life-world of the patient. The therapeutic slant is similar to that of humanistic and phenomenological approaches to psychotherapy, which aim to achieve more than behavioural change. Patients may be encouraged to examine the meaning of their experiences and to look upon events and relationships from different angles so as to become more aware of fixed and possibly unconscious patterns of behaviour. North American psychotherapist Donald Moss offers his own understanding:

> Phenomenological psychotherapy is never content with a simple change in behavior. Rather, the patient is invited to see his or her world in a different light, to discover a novel perspective on life and relationships, and to recapture a sense of wonder in a fresh and vital way of perceiving. This transformed perception and interpretation of life events becomes the avenue for practical modifications in behavior and relationships.[5]

When both light and shadow are recognised, patients are better able to deal with the hidden issues that may be influencing their health and wellbeing. Holistic approaches to healing aim to facilitate a deepening awareness of how our physical, mental and social activities can affect our state of health. A practitioner of homoeopathy offers her own contribution:

> *There are two things I'm looking at. I'm looking at the acute complaint . . . But beyond that, I'm looking at what will help the system heal itself, and strengthen it. Well, how can the immune system be strengthened? And so we give medicines that work on the entire constitution of the person, and look at not just the physical array of symptoms, or the physical characteristics, but also the emotional or mental characteristics of the person.*

This quote describes an approach that seeks to restore not only the body's physiological balance, but also to address psychological issues that are generally not the concern of general practice biomedicine. The acute or presenting symptoms are certainly given needed attention. But the task of healing also calls the practitioner to reflect upon the mental and emotional realities in their patients' lives.

For the homoeopath quoted above, psychosomatic medicine is more than an interesting theoretical aside. It is part of the essential foundation of authentic and responsible physicianship. All elements of our nature, not just the physical, must be brought to the task of resolving the disharmony that manifests as illness and disease. The patient's self-healing capacity is to be activated, and his or her physiological defences are to be strengthened.

Strengthening the patient

Our homoeopath goes on to describe her understanding of how these high aims are to be achieved:

> I'm looking at trying to match the person that I'm seeing and all of their life history and their problems, with what I know about these medicines. I'm trying to get them one which would fit best and to which their vital force would resonate, so that if they're given that medicine, the vital force then somehow corrects itself. It's like they're just given that tiny little push in the right direction . . . and some people have said that it's roughly analogous to a vaccine principle. But it's really much more refined.

Here we gain some insight into how the holistic healing intention is expressed and interpreted in homoeopathic practice. One of the more unusual aspects of the homoeopathic modus operandi is the fact that individual medications are not prescribed according to a given or specific diagnosis. Three patients with the same biomedical diagnosis may well receive three different homoeopathic medicines that are selected as much on the basis of the patient's personal characteristics and life history as on their actual presenting symptoms.

Nor can the medicines used by homoeopaths be categorised according to the norms of pharmacology. Their mode of action cannot be interpreted according to known pharmacodynamic principles. The stronger-acting homoeopathic potencies contain no physical substance other than lactose, or milk sugar, or a mixture of alcohol and water. Yet such medicines are said to carry influences capable of interacting with the energetic processes that animate our physical bodies. Traditional Chinese medicine similarly describes energies that course through and influence the activities of our physical bodies. Such conceptual systems clearly lie well beyond the present boundaries of science and the physicalist paradigm upon which biomedicine is based.

Implicit in this homoeopath's understanding is the notion that our human natures are a living Gestalt that can be in a state of harmony or disharmony. Homoeopathic medicines are said to affect the entire patterning of vital energies that sustain our being. They represent energetic templates that can stimulate the self-corrective tendencies that are part of our natures. She invokes the principle of resonance in order to explain how such 'impossible' medicines may do their work.

Underlying the homoeopathic approach is a pattern of history-taking and clinical engagement that consciously explores the physical, social and psychological dimensions of the patient. As consultations proceed, patients will inevitably become more aware of aspects of their lives that may previously have been dismissed, forgotten or over-shadowed. This in itself will increase their personal understanding of background circumstances that may be contributing to their condition.

Typically, homoeopaths view their patients and their conditions in energetic rather than physico-chemical terms. They view their mission in terms of a radical activation of corrective and healing influences. If the job is well done, patients may well experience more than a simple clearing of symptoms. She continues:

> When healing takes place, it might be that the person hasn't got a very well defined physical complaint when they come but they just want to enhance their general health. And you can often just feel it around them that their energy has changed after taking the medicine. It's just from practice that you get more sensitive to those energy fields. I don't see them myself but I feel them very strongly.

Not only does she make use of 'medicines' that contain no pharmacologically active substance, but she further reports that the effects of such medicines may be tangible to both the patient and those who administer them. And she fully accepts that others among her colleagues are capable of visually perceiving their patients' energy fields, and can thereby directly monitor their state of vitality.

Despite their sometimes heretical status, both homoeopathy and acupuncture have won the support of numerous patients throughout the world, who clearly benefit from their use. This points to a need to broaden the conceptual and interpretive framework of scientific medicine, an issue that will be taken up further in the following chapter.

On shamanic empowerment

Not all patients are driven to participate in their own health-making. Many believe it is best to leave matters relating to personal health in the hands of their doctor, who has both the knowledge and authority to provide whatever guidance may be necessary. Others may have difficulty in accepting the notion that their own behaviours contribute significantly to a failure of their health or to an increased proneness to disease. Regarding such matters, Fritjof Capra has commented:

> The first step in this kind of self-healing will be the patients' recognition that they have participated consciously or unconsciously in the origin and development of their illness, and hence will also be able to participate in the healing process. In practice, this notion of patient participation, which implies the idea of patient responsibility, is extremely problematic and is vigorously denied by most patients.[6]

It is difficult to apply the principles of holistic medicine across the board. A broad acceptance of holistic medicine will necessarily require a broader acceptance of the holistic basis of life, which holds that each of us represents an integral confluence of material, mental and living influences in constant interaction with each other and with the world.

In order to understand how holism can find expression in the context of healing, it may be helpful to review the role that the shaman serves in traditional cultures. Shamanic healers are generally called upon when one believes that their life is in disarray or that their life energies have been somehow vitiated by unknown forces. The shaman sets about to identify influences in another's life-world that may be causing disturbance, disorder or disease. The primary role of the shaman is 'to mediate power in order to restore balance and harmony'.[7] Such a restoration will then enable the patient to regain autonomy and equilibrium. British psychologist Helen Graham describes one of the major elements in the shamanic approach to healing:

> Whereas in the modern sense illness is an external agent entering the body, something to be destroyed or protected against, in the shamanic system it is loss of personal power that allowed the intrusion in the first place. All shamanic treatment therefore emphasises augmenting the power of the sick person, and only second-arily in counteracting the power of the illness-producing agent, which is seen to constitute a threat to health only when a person's protective mantle develops a weakness. Accordingly, the shaman does not work exclusively in the context of disease. His aim is the restoration of balance.[8]

The shaman seeks to empower patients through connecting deeply with their life-world. In traditional societies, this is achieved by the use of story, ritual chanting, gesture and movement, and invocation. In Western contexts, encouraging patient self-knowledge through conscious education and inner reflection may serve similar ends.

The power mediated by the shaman needs to be understood in terms appropriate to the culture and context within which the healing engagement occurs. The Siberian shaman may identify the source of her power as ancestral; the faith healer as the action of the Holy Spirit or the intervention of disembodied entities; the *curandero* of Central America as the power within such agents as *Banisteriopsis* vines or *Psilocybe* mushrooms. The activation of such qualities as imagination, creative visualisation and vitality in patients may be understood in a similar light.[9]

Personal power is an amalgam of many dimensions. Its presence is reflected in such qualities as self-knowledge, strength of will and the capacity for discipline and self-regulation. It finds expression in such attributes as autonomy, resilience, vitality and social competence. The holistically sensitive physician helps patients in the task of identifying those influences that may have contributed to a weakening of defences or a lowering of reserves. The knowledge gained through this process enables patients to actively increase their health and decrease their susceptibility to sickness or disease.

The way we live

Once we understand that the way we live affects our state of health, our perception of the nature of disease may undergo a change. Illness may no longer be viewed as a random or mysterious assault by unknown forces upon our being, but might be understood as an often avoidable and occasionally inevitable consequence of the way we that live our lives.

Left to its own devices, the world will continue to draw us towards a life of endless diversion and equally endless consumption, whether it be through the fiery intensity of bourbon, the pungent fragrance of tobacco or the sweet delights of sugar-laden confectionery. Such joys may well become an established part of our pattern of living in adult life. To have knowledge of what is useful and what is potentially harmful does not guarantee that we will necessarily choose the former. The multitude of cigarette smokers are testament to this truth.

We are often caught up in behaviours we know to be harmful, even when confronted by evidence of their direct effects upon our own health and that of our families and friends. The real question of how to improve our health and resistance to sickness may rest with more deeply rooted issues such as personal motivation and empowerment of the will to change than with pharmaceutical prescriptions or suggestions of what we should or should not do. A naturopath addresses this dilemma:

It's a matter of not only prescribing remedies and changing diets. It's changing habits, it's changing attitudes. Quite often it's the incorrigible person, not the incurable disease, as we've heard expressed in this profession. And old habits die hard. A lot of people are quite happy to continue on in their lifestyle regardless of the consequences.

Apart from the personal choices available to us in matters related to our individual lifestyle, we are also often obliged to live and work within situations that may subtly undermine our health. A number of industries work around the clock, meaning that their workers do the same. Many people in the developed world spend most of their working days under the fluorescent lights of air-conditioned buildings. And many commuters spend one or two hours daily contending with the snail-pace ordeal of the morning and afternoon peak-hour rush on crowded freeways or in the cramped carriages of urban rail systems.

It is worth contemplating what the social and economic consequences might be of a widespread reaction to the potentially damaging effects of such ways of living. But few have the freedom to get off the treadmill. The political and economic organisation of Western society is so structured that we often feel obliged to maintain high levels of income or risk losing our economic security and way of life, even if this comes at a significant cost to our health and personal freedom.

Although we have comfortably adapted to ways of living that are far removed from the fresh air and physical activity integral to human livelihood for thousands of years, we continue to be influenced by natural cycles that were established over evolutionary periods. Medical philosopher Rene Dubos reminds us that our wellbeing is conditioned not only by the state of our bodies and minds, but also by the rhythms and cycles of the natural world:

Health depends upon a state of equilibrium among the various internal factors that govern the operations of the body and the mind; this equilibrium in turn is reached only when man lives in harmony with his external environment. Ancient medicine never achieved an understanding of the nature of the forces controlling the internal environment; indeed, this knowledge began to develop barely a century ago. But one finds in the Hippocratic writings many details concerning the influence that the external environment exerts on human affairs.[10]

The holistic approach accepts that we are not infinitely adaptable beings capable of accommodating all the impositions and excesses of the humanly engineered environments within which many of us live out our lives. There are natural limits. Our capacity to maintain homoeostasis in the face of continuous stresses and excesses may eventually be broken. The task of the physician is not only to identify pathological changes in our internal operations and offer appropriate interventions, but equally to recognise when such deleterious changes may derive from imbalances in the way we live. A naturopath offers further insight:

> It's this whole concept that health has got something to do with a doctor coming along or a practitioner of any kind coming along to fix things. The whole fixing thing. There's no such thing as fixing. It's a political thing too. It's a kind of sociological and political thing because this lack of attention to health and rest and having a balanced life is reflected through the entire society. People don't convalesce their illnesses. They don't go to bed with their flus and what-have-you. There's a kind of fascism in the workplace which doesn't allow that. Treat your small illnesses with respect and you won't develop, as soon, the large ones that kill you.

This reflection may be labelled home-spun wisdom, but it affirms an obvious truth regarding the widespread cultural dismissal of signals that call us to reflect on what is happening in our lives. Ignoring the effects of constant stress and chaotic lifestyles may cause our self-regulating systems to break down and our vital energies to progressively decline.

This quote shows an awareness that the political economy of the workplace will often override the needs of the individual. The naturopath observes that the longer-term neglect of such needs may manifest as a progressive weakening of the body's defences, a lowering of vital reserves, and an increased proneness to the so-called diseases of civilisation which represent major sources of mortality in the West. Ivan Illich has similarly pointed to the folly of ignoring the nature of a social and economic system that may be inherently damaging to many of those who enable it to be sustained:

> The fundamental reason why these costly [medical] beaurocracies are health-denying lies not in their instrumental but in their symbolic function: they all stress delivery of repair and maintenance services for the human component of the megamachine, and criticism that proposes better and more equitable delivery only reinforces the social commitment to keep people at work in sickening jobs.[11]

We all crave simple solutions. When they are found, they can be a true godsend. But the holistic approach necessarily includes not only the patient and their symptoms, but also the total context within which we live, and move, and have our being. The task of healing, though directed primarily towards the patient, must eventually include a commitment to the healing of social, economic and environmental pathologies. The big question, of course, is how this is to be achieved.

Igniting the healing power

The word 'healing' itself means different things to different people. For some, it signifies a form of recovery from illness and disease that has been mediated by psychic or spiritual forces. Jesus of Nazareth is the quintessential healer in this regard. In Corinthians I, the power to heal is described as one of the gifts of the Holy Spirit. The term healer is similarly associated with the laying on of hands and with notions of psychic projection or spiritual intercession. We also speak of the healing of wounds or of broken bones, and of the healing properties of certain plants.

Medical orthodoxy, however, has tended to regard the terms 'healer' and 'healing' as somehow tainted by connotations of mysticism or charlatanism. Yet the healing process, in its essential meaning, points strongly towards the activation and strengthening of an inherent capacity of living systems for self-repair and restoration. To be cured of a condition is to be freed of the symptoms or discomforts that characterise that condition. To be healed, however, implies a transformative process whereby the individual has been made 'whole' once again.

Healing is not something done to another by a person or a drug. It is an attribute of all living systems. Although some aspects of the human organism and human functioning may be viewed in machine-like terms, the processes of repair and self-renewal are as living flames that burn within us, continually transforming our embodied nature.

The cells that make up our body are continuously turned over in a process of breakdown and repair. Our skin is constantly shed while new cells form to replace it. The cells lining the stomach and digestive system are renewed every few days. White blood cells are replaced two or three times monthly, while four generations of red blood cells are recycled each year. Such processes are largely outside of our conscious control. They are part of the mysterious ability of living systems to grow, to repair and to regenerate themselves.

The human organism is infused by powerful healing forces whose activity can be released or enhanced through the mediation of an understanding practitioner. An osteopath reflects:

I think of myself not as a healer—I'd never describe myself as a healer—but as someone who has a tremendous interest in what constitutes a healing process, and an explorer of means to get that healing process working . . . But if things change,I would regard myself as no more than catalytic. And to every person involved in health care, they'd do well to look to their curiosity and questioning and doubt and to see in fact how very, very little anybody knows about the processes that we're talking about.

This comment subtly expresses the osteopathic principle that the body has an innate capacity to heal itself. That capacity for self-healing can be enhanced by the effects of sensitively applied structural correction. This osteopath distances himself from the suggestion that he is the source of the healing power that mediates the patient's recovery, and instead points to the essential mystery of the healing process itself.

The activation or reinforcement of an innate healing force is a therapeutic objective common to many of the modalities of complementary medicine, though often expressed in different ways.

Naturopathy: vitality, toxicity and regeneration

Naturopathic medicine is based on three principles. The first is that of vitalism, which holds that we are animated by a coherent life force that regulates and governs the growth, repair and regeneration of the body and its diverse systems. This near-universal principle has, in the European tradition, been called the *spiritus vitae*, or spirit of life, a term often used by Paracelsus and others of his time, and the *vis medicatrix naturae*, or the healing power of nature.

The second principle is that of toxicity, in which it is believed that the accumulation of toxins from dietary and environmental sources will have an adverse effect on health. This principle has been held by a number of traditions throughout history. The Greek historian Herodotus records how the periodic use of enemas and dietary restriction were part of the public health methods advocated by Egyptian doctors.[12] The Book of Leviticus in the Old Testament recommends a system of hygiene and dietary regulation for the benefit of the tribes of Israel. And apocryphal sources suggest that the Essene communities made use of ritual fasting and colonic cleansing to purify both body and spirit.[13] In more recent times, hygienists such as Bernard Jensen and Max Gerson have confirmed the potential benefits of periodic dietary restriction and colonic cleansing to clear the body of accumulated toxins.[14]

The third principle is that of regeneration, which suggests that the body can be actively renewed, both physiologically and biochemically. Naturalistic systems of medicine consciously take on the task of bodily regeneration and the strengthening of organ systems, known as *trophorestoration* as part of their therapeutic mission. A cultural precedent for this therapeutic goal exists in Ayurvedic medicine. *Rasayana* represents one of the eight divisions of Ayurveda, and concerns itself primarily with regeneration and rejuvenation. The practices of fasting, dietary restriction, massage, breathing exercises and yoga practice, and the use of herbal and mineral medicines form the essential modalities of this specialty area of Indian medicine.[15] Within the Western tradition, European alchemy sought to achieve similar ends through the preparation and use of mineral and herbal medicines. And the hygienist tradition seeks to attain physiological regeneration through fasting and dietary regulation.[16]

These three principles inform the distinctive therapeutic aims of naturopathic medicine. Life force and vitality are to be actively augmented, and influences that may obstruct or limit their activity are to be minimised. Accumulated metabolic wastes are to be cleared by the conscious elimination of toxins from both dietary and environmental sources, and through the stimulation of the body's own detoxifying mechanisms. And the body's restorative capacities are to be activated through the use of supportive medication, attention to patterns of exercise and rest, and dietary regulation. Such approaches serve to increase one's physiological reserves and thereby enable one to better deal with the inevitable stresses of life, and to slow down the degenerative processes usually associated with ageing.

The therapeutic goals of naturopathic medicine differ significantly from those of biomedicine, which aim primarily to provide rapid and effective treatment of symptoms associated with sickness and disease through the use of drugs and surgery.

Medicine and regeneration

Certain human disorders cannot be cured by any system of medicine and can only be controlled, if at all, through constant and ongoing medication. A number of endocrine and neurological conditions fall within this category. Many hereditary disorders and the longer-term consequences of such conditions as congestive heart failure, emphysema and end-stage kidney failure are similarly beyond restoration.

It has been claimed that 'naturopaths have questionable expectations that the body can overcome profound degenerative diseases'.[17] But a growing literature reports that the life-long prescription of powerful drugs for symptom control in chronic degenerative diseases such as arthritis, circulatory disorders and heart disease may not be the only effective therapeutic approach.

In the late 1970s, Australian physician Richard Taylor presciently suggested, 'It would indeed be ironic if the solution to coronary artery disease was the conversion of hospitals into gymnasia.'[18] By the mid-1990s, American medical researcher Ken Pelletier was to confirm the usefulness of non-orthodox methods for dealing with the latter-day epidemics of late-onset diabetes, osteoporosis, hypertension, hypercholesterolaemia and the age-related loss of cognitive function that poison the end-days of many within our technological civilisation. He observed:

> Every one of these supposedly inevitable declines can be slowed, halted and even reversed, according to a growing body of both animal and human research. There is abundant research that diet and exercise can remedy impaired carbohydrate metabolism and insulin intolerance as well as osteoporosis. In fact, research indicates that physically active older men have an ability to metabolise blood sugar identical to that of young athletes. Likewise, programs that work with people to improve memory, recall and intellectual skills such as reading have been shown to reverse mental deterioration in as few as five sessions.[19]

Drugs certainly alleviate the symptoms of many of the chronic degenerative conditions. But they are not the only approach available to any prepared to work closely with patients in programs based on the augmentation of life energies, detoxification of the body through hygienic and eliminative methods, and the activation of regenerative forces through mobilising physical and mental reserves. A practitioner of naturopathic medicine offers his own view:

> The latter part of the twentieth century has seen planned redundancy in just about everything. Cars, white goods, everything has a limited life. These are planned to go wrong. We understand that it's a part of the cycle of things. But the human body is different. We've got to get back to the potential to expand and grow and regenerate. Whereas everything else decays, the body has the capacity to regenerate. And if we can get them to focus on that model and get away from the experiences of the world around them, then they can change their thinking. You can't change their chronological age, but you can certainly change their biological age. So a person might be sixty years of age but can have the regenerated body of a forty-five year old.

This comment raises a number of important issues. It challenges the dominant cultural view that progressive loss of function and gradual decline are an inevitable part of the ageing process. Although he does not spell out the details, it is clear that this naturopath accepts that physiological rejuvenation is not only a valid therapeutic aim, but a realisable goal.

The problem is not so much how it is to be achieved, or what methods should be used, but rather how to enlist the active participation of patients in such a project.

Regenerative medicine is a therapeutic possibility that is only now beginning to enter the language of Western scientific medicine. But it is already part of the language of naturopathic medicine. Many practitioners seek to communicate that language to their patients in ways that encourage them to realise the possibility for themselves. Such approaches call for an act of choice on the part of the patient, who may need to make major changes in their behaviour or way of life. The physician or practitioner can communicate the potential for bodily regeneration that is available; but ultimately, it is the patient who must cross the Rubicon.

Extending the boundaries

The huge successes of biomedicine in such areas as infant mortality, infection control and the use of powerful diagnostic technologies created an intellectual and moral environment that virtually demanded compliance with an approach whose efficacy was superior to anything that had preceded it. As the limitations of biomedicine progressively came to light, and as alternative approaches became more readily available and culturally acceptable, other perspectives regarding the nature of health and disease began to enter the picture.

We find ourselves at a time where the boundaries that previously defined the nature of 'acceptable' medicine have noticeably softened. We are witnessing a broadening tolerance towards views that only a few short decades ago would have been considered heretical. While some argue over the tenability of certain philosophies of healing, others appear to adopt a more pragmatic 'wait and see' attitude, and observe for themselves the effects of therapeutic approaches that differ from those endorsed by Western scientific medicine.

No one system has all the answers. Each has its own distinctive qualities and peculiar strengths. The work ahead requires a careful and sensitive appraisal of those qualities and strengths so that patients may better choose, or be better guided towards, approaches that will enable their needs to be more fully realised. Holistic approaches, by their nature, welcome complexity and diversity. They fully acknowledge the revolutionary importance of scientific understandings of the body and its workings that have emerged in recent centuries. But they also acknowledge the profound mystery carried within life itself, and accept that mind and consciousness are both implicate and influential in the life of the body.

A practitioner of traditional Chinese medicine describes his own approach:

If somebody says, 'Well, what would you do in this situation?', I usually say, 'Well, it's probably not particularly relevant what I would do, but given the situation and my nature I'd probably go in this direction. But there are these other possibilities as well, and what you need to do is to decide for yourself what's the appropriate thing for you to do.' Now, I mean, 'do' is probably too strong a word, because sometimes I find that really the understanding of the nature of crisis or of disharmony or whatever words we choose to use is in itself the healing process, because it gives people the confidence to let go and let the healing process actually move on a few more turns.

This comment points towards the delicacy of interaction through which a patient is encouraged to reflect upon both the nature of their condition and the nature of the healing process itself. It also highlights the intimate connection between healing and consciousness.

From the holistic perspective, the patient must become more than a passive recipient of treatments. Their own understanding of the condition itself and its possible origins, and their awareness of the choices available to them, will no doubt have a direct influence on the healing process. At times, even the most carefully selected medication and skilfully applied treatment will not eliminate painful or debilitating symptoms. One's mental and emotional attitude may then make the difference between whether one accepts the prospect of ongoing pain or limitation with mindful resignation, or whether one gives way to passivity or despair. An active and informed acceptance of limitation enables one to remain receptive to other approaches that may lighten the burden, or deepen the meaning of the experience.

Recovering the art

Some amongst us are afflicted early in life by major diseases such as leukaemia and epilepsy. Others may develop such conditions as diabetes or high blood pressure during what would otherwise be their more productive years. The longer we live, the greater the likelihood that we will encounter the limitations associated with ageing and chronic degenerative change. When medicines are no longer curative, and serve only to provide transient symptomatic relief, the role of the physician necessarily changes. More may be needed than the monitoring of blood readings and a periodic review of medication.

An integrated medicine must work not only with the needs of the body but with those of the soul. Although our bodies may be viewed in machine-like terms, and treated accordingly, they are also vehicles of our human consciousness and an experiencing self. A failed pregnancy may, according to the former view, be seen as a medical condition for which decisive action needs to be taken. Such action may include a thorough cleansing of the interior of the womb through curette procedure and the prescription of a course of strong antibiotics to ensure freedom from possible associated infection. Yet the same event may also represent the collapse of a dream, and an agonising search for the meaning of such a loss in the life of a young couple. It is not only the woman's womb that needs healing. Meredith McGuire observes:

> Adherents of alternative healing . . . often have radically different notions of what needs to be healed, what they consider to be a healing, and how healing takes place. Furthermore, their interpretations of illness embody their attempts to deal with the problems of *meaning* that are linked with illness, pain, suffering and death. The issue of meaning is generally not addressed by the dominant medical system, but in many alternative systems it is central. Why do people suffer? Why do people get sick despite preventive measures? Why do good people have troubles and bad people appear to flourish? Why do some people die 'before their time'?[20]

The holistic approach does not shy away from such issues. Nor does it divide the role of the practitioner into technical and non-technical compartments. In some ways, it calls for a re-awakening of the traditional ideal of the universal doctor, the priest-doctor, the shaman-healer who has assimilated a knowledge of both the physical and non-physical worlds, who is competent in ministering to the needs of the body, alert to subtle causative influences in the patient's life-world, and sensitive to the role of mind in the healing process.

The actualisation of such possibilities is not the exclusive domain of any one system of medicine. More than anything else, it requires an openness to different ways of seeing the world and a willingness to support and at times guide patients in their own movement towards greater knowledge and self-reliance. The practice of medicine is potentially much larger than disease identification and symptom correction. Many patients would surely welcome the opportunity to participate in therapeutic programs that increase their vitality and powers of resistance. An osteopath voices this notion succinctly:

> For the patient of course, they'll get something, and they'll get Medicare rebates and they'll probably be reassured that they haven't got a major pathology, you know in terms of Pap smears, and an X-ray taken and a scan taken. But are they better? Have they progressed in themselves? Are they more healthy from having visited the doctor? I don't think the

patients get what they really need. They get some part of it, certainly the cutting edge. They find out they're not dying and they don't have a major pathology.

This reflection provides a quintessential statement of the therapeutic aims of holistic medicine. Reductionist medicine has largely realised its historical task of charting the minute details of human anatomy, physiology and bio-chemistry. It has similarly detailed the nature of pathological processes and the physical and chemical interventions that will help the organism to return to a state of equilibrium and freedom. In recent decades, this has translated into an ethos that defines good medicine as the capacity to carefully and accurately diagnose diseases, and to skilfully direct biomedical knowledge to the task of overcoming pathology and at least providing symptomatic or palliative relief where cure is not possible.

A medicine that focuses exclusively on the physical body and its treatment is necessarily incomplete, although it can mean the difference between life and death, limitation and freedom. The task confronting medicine today is that of broadening even further its field of operation. Although knowledge of the body and its diseases has been largely mastered, there is yet much work to be done in similarly mastering a knowledge of the nature of mind and of spirit, and of their influence upon the remarkable capacity of living systems for self-repair and regeneration.

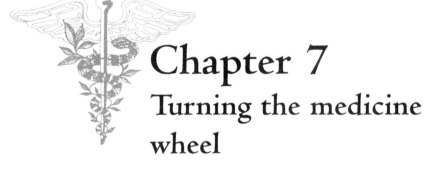

Chapter 7
Turning the medicine wheel
Between paradigms

Nothing that exists exists for its own sake; it exists for the sake of the whole.
Jean Gebser, 1949[1]

Far from constituting the pinnacle of human evolution, or the ultimate flowering of 'progress', the attitude of rationalism is an evolutionary dead end.
Georg Feuerstein, 1987[2]

The cultural dominance of biomedicine and its extraordinary successes have led many to believe it to be the one true medicine, the safe and effective medicine that has evolved out of the ages, superior in every way to everything coming before it and to the many other, lesser known, systems of medicine. Biomedicine has realised its present status through a commitment to what has become known as scientific method, a powerful method of inquiry aimed at generating new knowledge that can be codified, tested and transmitted to a professional community.

The key elements of scientific method are careful observation, rigorous measurement, experimentation and theory development. These elements have, in varying degrees, been part of the human endeavour to understand the phenomenal world throughout recorded history. This is reflected in the knowledge and skills used in architecture and building construction, astronomy and navigation, the discovery of medicinal agents and the practice of medicine.

Over the past century, the methods of science have been systematically applied to the study of the human body and its diseases. This has resulted in the new knowledge that underlies much of Western scientific medicine.

Biomedicine has developed out of a particular epistemological project. It is based, by and large, on the concepts of materialism, mechanism and rationality.

Holistic medicine fully accepts the validity of these concepts and the insights into the nature of the body and its diseases that they have given rise to. Holism by its nature also accepts that human life is influenced by factors other than those associated with materiality, mechanism and rationality. The role of mind in the creation of health and sickness, and the existence of an energetic or spiritual dimension associated with life represent elements of the holistic understanding for which acceptable epistemologies have yet to be developed.

Not entirely rationalist: Descartes and Newton

Scientific modernism is widely seen as one of the fruits of the methods developed by René Descartes and Isaac Newton during the seventeenth and eighteenth centuries. It is worth reflecting on both Descartes' and Newton's broader interests in order to better appreciate their relationship with the ideas and philosophies that have been posthumously ascribed to them.

René Descartes was born in France in 1596. As a young man, he was fascinated by the clarity, certainty and elegance of classical geometrical theorems. He wondered whether such certainty could be brought to bear on other aspects of human thought and endeavour. Putting aside the books and disputations that had characterised his early Jesuit upbringing, he began to seek out knowledge from direct experience and from the 'book of life'. He joined the Bavarian army as a soldier.

On the night of 10 November 1619, while sheltering from a severe winter in the city of Ulm, Descartes was profoundly shaken by three powerful dreams. These dreams ignited within him a sense of mission and destiny that were to drive him thereafter. On completion of his military training in 1623, he undertook a pilgrimage to the shrine of Our Lady of Loreto in Italy in gratitude for the insights gained that night in 1619. Although Descartes himself believed that the dreams had come from God, their influence upon him was later to be described as 'the most disastrous moment in the history of Europe'.[3]

Descartes set himself the task of creating a method of inquiry that would ensure all new knowledge would thereafter rest upon unshakeable foundations. This was to be established by applying his 'method of doubt'. That method was described in detail in his *Discourse on the Method of Properly Guiding the Reason in the Search of Truth in the Sciences*, written eighteen years after his illumination at Ulm. Central to Descartes' project was the separation of mind (*res cogitans*) from body (*res extensa*):

> Among the metaphysical theses developed throughout the *Meditations* is that mind and body have distinct essences; that the essence of thinking substance is pure thought/consciousness/awareness, while the essence of body is pure extension.[4]

Although he held near-mystical views of the nature of the mind, Descartes viewed the world, including living organisms, in mechanistic terms. He believed that the workings of complex systems could be understood through a systematic analysis of their individual components. This approach had a particularly strong influence on the methods that helped to empower the scientific revolution over the following two centuries.

The methods developed by Descartes were applied by a new generation of scientists who progressively retreated from spiritual or mystical interpretations of the world and its workings. The role of Divine influence steadily retreated as new knowledge led to greater powers of control and prediction. Ironically, Descartes himself maintained life-long friendships and correspondence with theologians, and lived and died as a devout Catholic.

Isaac Newton is remembered as the intellectual giant who gave to the world the *Principia Mathematica* in 1687. This work described, for the first time, revolutionary new methods of mathematical analysis. Newton's studies of the nature and interactions of light, and his discovery of the laws of gravity confirmed the extraordinary power of these methods. Newton showed conclusively that the physical universe operated according to immutable laws that, once known and understood, offered immense powers of control and predictability to those who understood them. He was a living vindication of Descartes' quest to find methods that would, once and for all, lead to a certain knowledge of truth.

Newton's genius was fed by an unyielding tenacity. A man of extraordinary discipline, he spent many of his younger years as a solitary observer of the night sky. He meticulously measured the movements of the planets through the fixed constellations, and the movements of the constellations through the seasons of the year. He made his own telescopes and experimented with various lenses, discovering that white light was composed of the various colours of the spectrum. Having been introduced to the works of Descartes, Kepler and Galileo while a student at Cambridge, Newton applied his genius to a series of investigations on the properties of light, the laws of motion and the movements of planetary bodies.

Between the lines, however, Newton gave over much of his formidable mental energy to wide-ranging alchemical investigations during his early years, and in an ongoing study of Church history and theology in his latter years. It is a curious fact that Newton's lesser known activities have been largely lost to history. American historian Betty Dobbs reflects:

The Newtonian world view, indeed, developed almost wholly on the basis of his successes in mathematics and physical science, so subtly and deeply colored the thoughts of succeeding generations that the fuller seventeenth-century context in which Newton's thought had developed was lost to view. Thus it became a curious anomaly—and one to be explained away—that Newton's studies in astronomy, optics and mathematics only occupied a small portion of his time. In fact, most of his great powers were poured out upon church history, theology, 'the chronology of ancient kingdoms', prophecy and alchemy.[5]

Although the rationalist paradigm that underlies much of Western science has long been associated with the names of René Descartes and Isaac Newton, one may well question whether either would be comfortable with the virtual elimination of the numinous in 'scientific matters' that has since been carried out in their name.

The great divide

Much of contemporary Western medicine is unlike anything that has ever preceded it. The immense body of medical knowledge accumulated through the collective efforts of countless healers over long periods of time was largely left behind once the new methods of science began to reveal their power.

Simple extracts of plants that had been used as medicines for thousands of years were replaced by a grain or two of purified alkaloids. Humoral diagnosis, based on the four elements of the ancients, was progressively put aside as new knowledge of anatomical pathology began to emerge. And spiritual or metaphysical interpretations of disease were deemed irrelevant after the discovery of disease-causing micro-organisms and the development of modern epidemiology.

Descartes' separation of the body from the mind, and Newton's demonstration that observation and measurement were the well-springs of certain knowledge, drove medicine ever deeper into materiality in its quest for power and control over human diseases. The new knowledge of the body and of its workings uncovered by early anatomists, physiologists and pharmacologists became the foundation upon which a powerful new institution began to take form.

By the first decades of the twentieth century, scientific medicine was well established throughout the West. Its practitioners acquired their knowledge through many years of intensive training in universities and hospitals. The new medicine was a dramatic medicine, a life-saving medicine, one capable of identifying disease with certainty and dealing decisively, if not with the disease itself, then with its distressing and painful symptoms through medication or surgery.

Reflecting on the ideas held by 'primitive' doctors and indigenous healers, medical historian Fielding Garrison was to declare in the late 1920s:

> Disease [was regarded] as something produced by a human enemy possessing supernatural powers, which he strove to ward off by appropriate spells and sorcery, similar to those employed by the enemy himself. Again, his own reflection in the water, his shadow in the sunlight, what he saw in dreams, or in an occasional nightmare from gluttony, suggested the existence of a spirit-world apart from his daily life and of a soul or *alter ego* apart from his body. In this way, he hit upon a third way of looking at disease as the work of offended spirits of the dead . . . These three views of disease are common beliefs of the lowest grades of human life.[6]

Having dismissed dreams as a by-product of disturbed digestion, and denying outright the existence of spiritual realities and the human soul, Garrison identified himself as a member of a new elite of healers whose knowledge and understanding had superseded the 'primitive' notions held by healers of other times and other cultures. Yet human nature does not necessarily conform to the Euclidean precision favoured by the scientific view of the world. Our consciousness and beliefs continue to be determined by cultural realities that are based on far more than science and rationality.

The urban shaman

American doctor Larry Dossey has recounted a memorable episode that occurred in the wards of the hospital in which he undertook his internship during the 1960s. A weakened and emaciated old man had been admitted to the hospital after having inexplicably lost more than 20 kilograms in weight over the previous six months. Cancer was immediately suspected, and the full range of pathology tests was ordered by his friend, a fellow intern who was in charge of the case. After two weeks of intensive investigations, the doctors were no closer to a diagnosis and the patient was growing steadily weaker. Dossey's friend said to the old man, 'You're dying and I don't know why.' His patient then confided that there was nothing that could save him, for a curse had been placed on him by a shaman. An enemy had secretly obtained a lock of the old man's hair, upon which the shaman had performed her magic. The old man had then been duly informed of the curse. His appetite had immediately dried up and he had begun to lose weight. His health steadily declined and he eventually ended up in hospital.

Dossey describes how he and his friend dealt with this dilemma. At midnight on the following Saturday, when few fellow staff members were present, Dossey roused the old man and quietly wheeled him through the darkened corridors to an examination room where Dossey's friend was waiting, sitting before a table. The only light in the room was a small blue flame flickering from an inflammable tablet placed on a metal tray. After a minute or two of complete silence, Dossey's friend ceremoniously rose from his seat and slowly approached the old man. Using a pair of stainless steel scissors, he cut a lock of hair from the old man's head. Fixing his eyes upon the old man, he lowered the hair into the flame intoning, 'As the fire burns your hair, the curse in your body is destroyed.'

After a further brief period of silence, they wheeled the old man out of the smoke-filled room and returned him to his bed. The transformation was immediate. The next morning, the old man ordered multiple serves of breakfast and continued to ask for extra helpings with each meal thereafter. Within a short time, both his strength and his weight began to return. As the old man left the hospital soon after, he smilingly thanked the two young doctors who had saved him.[7]

Human experience casts long shadows that are not so easily dispersed by new interpretations of the nature of the world, regardless of their power to explain phenomena or account for the mysterious. Looking at human disease and sickness in purely physical and mechanistic terms certainly provides us with clear and irrefutable stories of how diseases may arise and how they affect the body, but this is done at the cost of neglecting the many contexts from which we, as humans, draw meaning. The historical and cultural traditions within which we are raised can powerfully shape our view of the world and the forces within it.

A crisis in our own health, or in the health of a loved one, can draw forth many possible responses. As well as making use of whatever help scientific medicine can provide, many will also seek comfort and assistance through prayer. Places of worship such as Lourdes, Mecca, Varanasi and Medjugorje are regularly visited by many thousands of pilgrims who search for healing above and beyond the ministrations of the various medical professions. Such gestures do not necessarily reflect the actions of 'low grade' or 'primitive' minds. Rather, they affirm an understanding that we are moved by forces that have yet to be fully understood.

Beyond rationality: Jean Gebser

The transformations of medicine over the course of recorded history show that our understanding of the world can undergo quantum changes that affect both the way we think and the way we go about doing things. But we do not necessarily automatically discard the 'primitive' notions according to which we may have lived in the past. Although the power of analytical thought and our newly discovered capacity for rationality may have become signatures of the present technological age, these are not the sole determinants of our behaviour. The past is not so lightly shaken off.

Moved by the great contradictions lived out during the first half of the twentieth century, the Swiss cultural philosopher Jean Gebser sought to provide a perspective that offered some understanding of the dilemmas confronting the contemporary world. As a student of language and culture, Gebser cast his net far and wide in an attempt to discern the nature of the revolutions in consciousness that had led to the development of human rationality.

Gebser was more a generalist than a specialist, more an artist than a scientist. His ideas were drawn from the fields of literature, art, poetry, psychology and science. At the outbreak of World War II, he moved from France to Switzerland where he was befriended by the psychologist Carl Jung. Gebser found a ready audience at Jung's institute, where he lectured for many years.

Gebser's great fascination and interest lay in the development of human consciousness. He suggested that over the course of many thousands of generations, human consciousness has undergone a series of progressive mutations, each of which has radically altered our potential. He named these, in sequence, the archaic, the magical, the mythical and the mental modes of consciousness. Gebser also suggested that the mutation that informs the mental structure of consciousness, which is dominant today, has been active over the past 10 000 to 12 000 years. He suggests further that the rational mode of consciousness that has been so influential over the past 500 years represents the most recent, though not necessarily the most humane or balanced, development of the mental structure.

Writing in the late 1940s, Gebser suggested that humanity is presently undergoing another major mutation in consciousness; the mental structure, characterised by its philosophical and material accomplishments, is presently being infused by what Gebser has termed the integral structure, characterised by an increasingly holistic sensitivity and an intensification of spiritual energy. More will be said about this later in the chapter.

Gebser believed that earlier structures of consciousness, though apparently superseded, continue to exert their influence in subtle and often unconscious ways. Our present consciousness is conditioned not only by the newly emergent rationality that characterises the present age, but carries echoes of magical and mythical consciousness. Gebser's model provides a useful framework for understanding not only the contradictory currents that have moved the will to healing during different historical periods, but also those that presently govern relations between nations, between people and within ourselves.

In matters of health and sickness, we are moved by more than the massive cultural and institutional power exercised by scientific medicine. Despite the financial support of Western governments, the reassurance provided by rigorous medical education programs and the influence of public health campaigns, our responses to issues affecting our health continue to be visceral as well as rational, emotional as well as physical, philosophical as well as practical.

The deficiencies of a medicine founded largely upon materiality and rationality have awakened a growing realisation that there is more to the story. The movement towards holism in medicine seeks to identify and integrate elements that are presently generally neglected into a broader understanding. This may call not only for a reacquisition of medical skills and wisdom that have perhaps been prematurely discarded but, more importantly, for a renewed investigation of the nature and influence of the non-material and non-rational influences that are part of our lives.

Intuition and medicine

In recent centuries, the focus of medicine, the most human of all the sciences, has progressively shifted away from subjective human experience and turned increasingly towards objective signs and symptoms, and variables that can be controlled and limited. Fritjof Capra reflects on the consequences of this development:

> Ever since Galileo, Descartes and Newton our culture has been so obsessed with rational knowledge, objectivity and quantification, that we have become very insecure in dealing with human values and human experience. In medicine, intuition and subjective knowledge are used by every good physician, but this is not acknowledged in the professional literature, nor is it taught in our medical schools. On the contrary, the criteria for admission to most medical schools screen out those who have the greatest talents for practicing medicine intuitively.[8]

Capra recognises that good medicine can still be practised not according to the book. The accessibility, sensitivity and humanity of the physician may be as important in the healing process as objective diagnosis and strict adherence to medication schedules. Capra notes that in the actual clinical practice of medicine, regardless of modality, neither subjective knowledge nor intuition are entirely overridden. Holistic medicine sits comfortably with such considerations. Understanding the role of the patient's life-world, their emotional realities, their motivations and their limitations rests upon more than a knowledge of pathophysiology and access to high-tech diagnostics.

Capra also notes that gaining high scores in the hard sciences may not be the most appropriate basis for entry into the healing professions. Despite the fact that a number of medical schools have begun to incorporate elements of the liberal arts and humanities in their programs, biomedicine remains firmly grounded in scientific knowledge. The criteria for entry into medicine continue to turn upon one's performance in mathematics, chemistry and physics.

A naturopath reflects on the role of intuition in his own approach:

I see the boundaries of the paradigm from which medicine comes as being very narrow, very circumscribed. And I think the difference is that as natural therapists we have extended our horizons or our boundaries out a lot more, so that we are working perhaps on what we call intuitive levels, or using things that work in terms of clinical results. But we may not have actual explanations for them at this point in time.

For this practitioner the boundaries within which certainty has been painstakingly charted by scientific medicine can represent as much a source of limitation as of therapeutic power. He has an interest in influences that cannot be fully measured or quantified. These would include such notions as patient motivation and patient vitality. He speaks of working on intuitive levels, as well as making use of empirically effective strategies. This reflects an openness to therapeutic possibilities that transcend strictly pharmacological approaches to healing.

Changing paradigms

The influence of Cartesian dualism during the eighteenth and nineteenth centuries freed science from the problem of mind, and made matter (in the case of science) and the body in particular (in the case of medicine) the primary fields of investigation. The phenomenal world came to be understood through a study of its constituents. The mechanisms underlying the interactions and inter-relationships of those constituents were sought through experimentation, and interpreted through the prism of mathematical analysis.

Medical philosopher Lawrence Foss has observed that the principles of dualism, reductionism and determinism provided the basis for the explanatory strategies used in all scientific investigations. In the case of biomedicine, the disciplines of physics, biochemistry and molecular biology represent the foundational elements from which there emerged a progressive understanding of pathophysiology, the study of disease processes.[9]

Lawrence Foss raises the conundrum presented by numerous research findings in medical literature supporting the notion that activities of the mind can have an effect on the health of the body. He cites a five-year research study that was terminated six months before it was due to be completed because it overwhelmingly confirmed the benefits of psychological counselling on the progression of coronary heart disease. Yet this and many other studies, as Fritjof Capra has said, have 'failed to have a significant influence on mainstream medical thinking'.[10] Mind, human subjectivity and the nature of consciousness remain vast jousting grounds of conjecture.

The findings of such studies, together with the many 'anomalous' phenomena, including the placebo effect, that are associated with the healing process, cannot at present be satisfactorily accounted for by the paradigms underlying scientific medicine. The question of whether contemporary Western medicine adheres to a single paradigm or whether it is an aggregate of a number of differing paradigms is also fraught. One often hears of reductionist or holistic paradigms, materialist or energetic paradigms, and disease-oriented or health-oriented paradigms of medicine.

The term paradigm in itself may represent a further source of confusion. Social researcher Egon Guba comments:

> It is not surprising that most persons asked to define the term paradigm are unable to offer any clear statement of its meaning. I say it is not surprising because Thomas Kuhn, the person most responsible for bringing that concept into our collective awareness, has himself used the term in no fewer than 21 different ways.[11]

Guba himself has no problem with the ambiguity inherent in the term, as he believes that the concept remains useful precisely because of its indeterminate nature. Philosopher Carl Matheson offers his own reflection on the theme:

> There is considerable disagreement over the proper interpretation of the word 'paradigm'. At one extreme is a very narrow interpretation according to which a paradigm consists of a set of exemplars . . . At the other extreme a paradigm consists of an entire theoretical worldview . . . According to a third reading, which is orthogonal to the others, a paradigm is a fundamentally sociological entity, individuated and constituted by patterns of education and alliances . . . It is best to choose a fairly wide sense of the term.[12]

Regardless of the difficulty in nailing a precise meaning of the term, it continues to be used widely in discussions related to the various models underlying different forms of medical practice. Thomas Kuhn, the philosopher of science who first coined the term in 1962, has described the process whereby the particular understandings that underlie a given discipline can undergo major or even revolutionary change:

> The transition from a paradigm in crisis to a new one from which a new tradition of normal science can emerge is far from a cumulative process, one achieved by an articulation or extension of the old paradigm. Rather it is a reconstruction of the field from new fundamentals, a reconstruction that changes some of the field's most elementary theoretical generalizations as well as many of its paradigm methods and applications. During the transition period there will be a large but never complete overlap between the problems that can be solved by the old and the new paradigm . . . When the transition is complete, the profession will have changed its view of the field, its methods and the goals.[13]

This comment offers a useful means of interpreting the present difficulties confronting scientific medicine in relation to certain aspects of the phenomenon of healing, particularly those associated with mind–body healing. The problems are essentially paradigmatic, and reflect an essential inadequacy in the foundational elements underlying the practice of biomedicine. More holistic approaches to healing have, in recent times, contributed significantly to extending the 'view of the field' that may help to bring about a deeper understanding of realities that cannot presently be accommodated by the paradigms underlying scientific medicine.

Medicine and mind

The increasing community patronage of non-orthodox approaches to medicine during the latter half of the twentieth century presented a significant challenge to the cultural dominance of biomedicine. This challenge was at first largely dismissed. During the 1970s and 1980s, such developments began to be vigorously opposed in medical literature, and more broadly debated in political theatres and the media. More recently, however, a number of these approaches have been co-opted into the medical curriculum as units or programs in complementary or integrative medicine.

But the matter is not simply resolved by increasing the number of modalities that are considered acceptable, or by incorporating a few natural substances or unusual methods that have proven their efficacy, into the ways of biomedicine. The growing utilisation of complementary medicine throughout the Western world points to a need to address more deeply such issues as the foundations of human nature, the adequacy of reductionist epistemologies and treatment methods, and the role and influence of mind in both health and disease.

Acupuncture represents more than the insertion of stainless steel needles into selected points in the body. It embodies a profoundly holistic philosophy that places us within a sea of energy with which we are in constant interaction. The various herbal medicine traditions are more than sources of such therapeutic agents as *Echinacea angustifolia* or *Ginkgo biloba*. They place us within the matrix of life itself, sharing at a fundamental level the same living energy that drives a seed to its eventual expression as fragrant flower or towering tree. Osteopathy is more than one of the many modalities of physical medicine. It is founded upon an understanding that the human organism has a powerful, innate capacity for self-healing that can be mobilised by structural correction.

One of the more regretful consequences of the Cartesian project was the separation of mind from matter. The world of matter, the *res extensa* of Descartes, became the domain of scientific investigation. The physical world was seen to be subject to laws and mechanisms that could be uncovered and elucidated through the methods of science. That world included living organisms. The forces that maintained life were believed to be linked to physical and chemical processes that would in time be sufficiently understood to provide a comprehensive explanation of life itself. The *res cogitans*, or the world of mind, provided the means whereby rational intelligence could be directed towards understanding the nature of the material world.

In more recent times, our thoughts, emotions and mental activity have come to be viewed as epiphenomena, or the complex consequences of chemical reactions occurring within the *res extensa* of the brain and the central nervous system. This notion has been clearly articulated by Arthur Kornberg, Nobel Laureate in medicine and one of the founders of genetic engineering:

Can we come as close to understanding the mind and human behavior as we have metabolism? The first and formidable hurdle is acceptance without reservation that the form and function of the brain and nervous system are simply chemistry. I am astonished that otherwise intelligent and informed people, including physicians, are reluctant to believe that mind, as part of life, is matter and only matter . . . Brain chemistry may be novel and very complex, but it is expressed in the familiar elements of carbon, nitrogen, oxygen and hydrogen, of phosphorus and sulphur that constitute the rest of the body.[14]

A practitioner of traditional Chinese medicine expresses his own unease at the notion that either mind or human behaviour can be fully encompassed by the laws of chemistry and the laws that govern the transformations of matter:

> There has been a great silence in Western science about the things that we haven't been able to measure and quantify. And they are things like consciousness, awareness, the nature of being. And clearly people who are recognising and [are] aware of this great silence need to speak, and need to give people confidence to say: Yes. I am more than just my body.

This reminds us that the mystery of human nature encompasses more than the material domain. Materiality and rationality are only a part of the myriad influences that determine our lived experience. We can suffer as much through grief as we do from broken bones. Meaning resides as much in metaphor and symbol as in the identification and naming of disease processes. Although the fact of subjectivity may be a nuisance according to certain points of view, it nonetheless remains an integral part of human consciousness.

Not by bread alone

The reality of individual consciousness has not figured strongly in the biomedical paradigm. The elimination of subjectivity and the tethering of scientific endeavour to the 'objective' world, that part of the phenomenal world that can be observed and measured, has resulted in a neglect of much that gives individual human life its meaning. The model of the phenomenal world presented by Western science does not and cannot give the full picture. Economist and cultural reformer E.F. Schumacher offers a dose of wisdom:

> Science cannot produce ideas by which we could live. Even the greatest ideas of science are nothing more than working hypotheses, useful for the purposes of special research but completely inapplicable to the conduct of our lives or the interpretation of the world.[15]

Social forces are neither visible nor measurable, yet they condition our lived experience. Psychological and emotional tendencies do not have readily identifiable biochemical or physiological markers yet they colour and often determine our experience of the world. The spiritual realities that provide guiding principles for many among humanity are only passingly referred to, if at all, in any serious discussion of influences on health and disease.

Human consciousness is a variable phenomenon influenced by heredity, nurture, learning, experience and a number of drugs, among other things. As individuals, we often experience the same event in different ways. We may hear what we want to hear; we can have varying levels of understanding of the influence of childhood and adolescent experiences on the formation of our character or personality; our consciousness of even basic realities such as sound, taste or vision can vary from one person to another. And our consciousness of the more subtle dimensions related to energetic or spiritual reality is even more variable.

American nursing academic Dolores Krieger has introduced many within the nursing profession to an approach to healing that has become known as Therapeutic Touch. The term itself is a misnomer, for the technique does not involve any actual physical contact between practitioner and patient. This practice is based on an acceptance of the reality of a radiant or energetic body that substands and interpenetrates the physical body. Krieger developed her system of healing as a result of collaboration with Dora Kunz, an accomplished seer or visionary capable of perceiving the activity of luminous energies in and around the human body.[16]

Much of the healing that occurs in certain forms of shamanism, particularly those associated with the use of psychoactive drugs, is said to be mediated through the manipulation of luminous energies that become available to the shaman and often to fellow participants during healing rituals and ceremonies. Cultural anthropologist Terence McKenna reports on the role of luminous energies in certain shamanic rituals:

> Shamans, under the influence of potent monoamine oxidase-inhibiting, harmine- and tryptamine-containing *Banisteriopsis* infusions, are said to produce a fluorescent violet substance by means of which they accomplish all their magic. Though invisible to ordinary perception, this fluid is said to be visible to anyone who has ingested the infusion.[17]

Religious traditions of most cultures speak of luminosity and radiance as qualities associated with the presence of spiritual energy. And many of those traditions associate that spiritual energy with a potential for healing both body and mind.

Biomedicine is of necessity, a thoroughly secular profession. This is a direct consequence of its foundational relationship with scientific method and its largely materialist orientation. Such a secular role is fully consistent with the pluralism that characterises Western society. But over and above their formal university training, many practitioners of biomedicine hold religious and spiritual beliefs. Some are regular church-goers or practitioners of meditation. Individual practitioners remain free to quietly work according to their own understanding of what is possible.

As the boundaries of what is considered acceptable progressively broaden, we may begin to witness an increase in interest in both the nature of such energies and their potential application for the purposes of healing.

Life force

Many within complementary medicine sit comfortably with such notions as *energy*, *vitality* and *spirit* and their influence in the work of healing. The notion of a life force is central to the understanding of many practitioners of naturo-pathic medicine. A naturopath offers his own reflection:

> Life force I believe is innate in everyone. The Indians call it prana. We all have it, this vitality. Animal magnetism, other people call it. The ch'i, the Chinese call it. It's a force or a vitality that is partly, I believe, electromag-netic in nature. But it is expansive, it has the capacity to just grow and grow and to amplify. This can be turned up or turned down, like a dimmer on a light. By using the correct principles of living, I believe it can be amplified and turned up.

This comment reflects the inherent difficulty of dealing with experiences and concepts for which there is no common language. It is suggested here that the term life force points towards a phenomenon that has yet to be identified and investigated by medical science. This naturopath further suggests a close relationship between the state of the body and the quality of that life force. He believes that the human energy field can be made stronger by certain practices and 'by using the correct principles of living'.

Jan Smuts, who coined the term 'holism' in the 1920s, recognised early the difficulty of finding the right language to describe activities within living systems:

> Body-and-soul is the model or scheme on which both thought and science are based. There is an *anima* dwelling in a *corpus*, one entity living in close symbiosis with another. As Descartes formulated it, there is the *res cogitans* in the *res extensa*; there are two distinct separate *res* or entities, and the difficulties and contradictions arise from their mutual assumed interaction.
>
> The theory of Vitalism or the vital force seems simply to emphasise this dualism. But if we wish to overcome these difficulties and contradictions we have to probe more deeply than these popular views. We must get down to the tap-root from which the two apparent entities or substances have grown. The subject is most difficult and uncertain.[18]

Those difficulties and uncertainties continue into the present day.

An osteopath offers a serious-minded attempt to interpret the meaning of ch'i, a term used in traditional Chinese medicine to describe the energetic currents associated with living bodies:

Talking first of all about ch'i. It's not an it. It's a them. There is an enormous chemical soup and interchange of movement and heat and so on going through the body and all round the body in all sorts of different directions at all times, and to pick out the electrochemical or electro-magnetic aspect of that or to pick out the circulation of endorphins or whatever and say, 'Oh, this is what we are talking about, that's what we're talking about.' No. The idea of ch'i is a metaphor, an abstraction and a simplification of a way of perceiving some currents that are going on in that chemical soup if you like. And it's not an it. It's a them. It's a simplification of many things into one to try and make sense.

This quote suggests that the term *ch'i* points towards the energetic dimension of changes that may occur on a physiological or biochemical level. In this sense, he is far closer to Smuts' perspective than the naturopath quoted earlier. He notes that elements within these electromagnetic fields may be associated with the neural and chemical activity that are integral to metabolism. Whether such energetic manifestations represent a unified dynamic that encodes information reflective of functional aspects of the body and its organ systems is, however, another story.

It is well understood that heat represents the physical expression of electromagnetic vibrations in the infra-red region of the electromagnetic spectrum. In a similar way, the electrochemical changes associated with the transmission of neurologic impulses throughout the nervous and sensory systems may create their own subtle fluctuations that are reflected in the bioenergetic field associated with our living bodies. There is clearly more to the picture than flesh and blood. But our osteopath reserves judgement regarding the various interpretations of the nature and significance of these energies. He continues:

Saying ch'i energy or saying chakras or saying meridians, or auras, or astral-bodies and so on, are simplifications, in order to try and make something explicable in a more concrete form when you perceive it, and to have a language of talking to other people about it. In another sense, they are actually metaphorical perceptions in that we are not ever perceiving the real.

This comment reflects the inherent difficulty of articulating the nature of perceptions that may vary between one individual and another.

The fact that widely diverse cultures have given linguistic expression to perceptions of energy through the use of such terms as ch'i, prana, chakras, meridians, spirit and auras points strongly towards their universality. The osteopath quoted above views these terms as metaphors for the intangible. With no common language, interpretation remains idiosyncratic. With no material substance, there is nothing to grasp and hold. The finger can only point to the moon.

A practitioner of Western herbal medicine offers his own view of the relevance of such considerations in the clinical setting:

> I believe that there is an energy. But it's not something that I focus on. It's not something I will ever talk about, but I believe that there is an underlying factor there. I believe it takes many, many years of clinical exposure to start to understand it, let alone work with it. I feel that component is there but it's not something which I particularly focus on. I believe that as an individual practitioner, within an individual practitioner's model, it may have some importance. But I believe that its importance tends to be overrated. The knowledge is useful. But I don't believe that it's a very important aspect of it.

This herbalist acknowledges the existence of an energy that can be used for healing purposes, but is reluctant to discuss the matter further in the clinical context. There exists no scientifically acceptable paradigm or conceptual model that comfortably accommodates such possibilities. Nor is there a common language through which these ideas can be expressed. Yet this practitioner accepts that some practitioners can and do utilise such notions in their daily work.

As with our earlier quoted osteopath, such considerations are not central to his work as a clinician or as an educator. Nor can they be said to be central to the practice of holistic medicine. But an acceptance of the reality of such energies, that are nowhere addressed within the discourse of biomedicine, creates a certain tension between the principles that can be openly acknowledged as the basis of one's healing activities, and those that remain unspoken.

Beyond the margins

During the 1960s, American psychiatrist Shafica Karagulla conducted a series of depth interviews with individuals who exhibited what she called 'higher sense perception'. Dora Kunz, who provided much of the insight that enabled Dolores Krieger to develop the methods of therapeutic touch, was among her interviewees.

Karagulla also interviewed a number of medical practitioners as part of her study. Some spoke of perceiving energy fields in and around their patients' bodies; others of being able to relieve acutely ill patients by placing their hands over the affected areas. One practitioner claimed the ability to look directly into the body and observe the activity of its various organ systems in order to determine the presence or absence of pathology. Another formed her tentative diagnoses on the basis of the nature and quality of the energy fields she perceived around her patients. Most interestingly, all of these respondents tended to hold silence both with their patients and their peers regarding their abilities, preferring rather to use conventional diagnostic procedures in order to validate their own observations and intuitions:

> Almost without exception they kept quiet about their unusual talents because they feared any mention of such things might hurt their professional standing. In most cases each had felt that perhaps he [or she] was alone and peculiar in this regard. [19]

Those interviewed were not part of the so-called lunatic fringe of alternative medicine, but were competent and fully qualified practitioners of biomedicine. And despite the fact that their own perceptions did not conform to what are considered normal or valid sources of knowledge from the scientific perspective, they continued to make use of their observations in their professional life. At a more personal level, however, the cost of inhabiting such a perceptual world contributed to a degree of alienation from their colleagues, and a loss of freedom to discuss among peers their own observations for fear of estrangement and possible ridicule.

One of the more interesting aspects of Karagulla's study is the fact that virtually every respondent offered a differing description of their observations. Such a situation represents a methodological nightmare in terms of generating a consistent and reproducible charting of the perceptual terrain inhabited by those able to directly perceive the subtle energetic currents associated with living processes. Karagulla's study represents an early entry into an area that has for too long been either denied, neglected or quietly pursued on an individual level.

Another naturopath furthers the discussion:

> Within the naturopathic arena, there will be those whose frontier will continue to evolve. And so what I believe will happen in the future, is that natural therapists of whatever persuasion are going to go more and more into energy medicine. It's as if there is always a group within the natural medicine arena that remains the frontier band, even though some of the guard may be absorbed into [orthodox] medicine, if that makes sense. So

there will be those that really start to work purely at an energetic level. They'll basically just look at a person, be able to see energy imbalances, and from their own mind powers start to create changes.

This naturopath is not alone in his projections. American sociologist Meredith McGuire comments on similar ideas expressed by respondents in her own study of non-orthodox approaches to healing:

Many respondents felt that their alternative healing approaches were actually ahead of medical science. They were sure that when it gained the ability to tap such phenomena, medical science would vindicate most of these alternatives. They believed that science was only beginning to discover the truth of what their belief system had told them all along.[20]

It is clear that there are many healers operating outside the framework of biomedicine who both accept the reality of an energetic dimension to human nature, and accept that certain individuals are capable of perceiving and interpreting such energies, and of intervening at a purely mental or volitional level. Such notions fall well beyond the boundaries of the current paradigms that inform biomedical understanding.

Medicine and energy

Material observations will respond to material interventions. An altered blood chemistry can be remedied by the use of material medicines, such as iron supplements for anaemia. But when one begins to speak in energetic rather than material terms, new possibilities begin to enter the picture.

A homoeopath respondent offers her own thoughts on the conceptual dilemma confronting practitioners who work from an energetic perspective:

I think that things like Kirlian photography are touching the edge of it. There is the work of Rupert Sheldrake who has talked about morphic fields and morphic resonance. I think he's at the forefront of the cutting edge of science. I think that it is going to come because to me it is so real that it has to. It's just that science, the paradigm that we have at the moment, doesn't incorporate these concepts or these understandings of subtler energies, subtler realms.

Neither homoeopaths nor acupuncturists are necessarily capable of directly perceiving energy fields associated with the body. Yet practitioners of each approach aim to bring about a primary corrective transformation in such subtle energies in patients. These approaches are based on a view of living systems that is very different to that described by the biomedical paradigm.

The quote above mentions such recent developments as electrophotography, developed by Russian scientist Semyon Kirlian, and the challenging theories of Rupert Sheldrake as invitations for serious-minded investigations of these areas. Kirlian photography in many ways represents a technology whose day has perhaps come and gone too quickly. Yet much of the work done in the 1970s confirmed its potential usefulness as a research tool for the investigation of biological and intentional energies.

Apart from the sheer beauty of many of the images produced by the technique, Kirlian photography offers a means of creating images which confirm that *something* changes in such activities as deep meditation, spiritual healing and active visualisation. The nature of that something, however, remains elusive, as there are no commonly acceptable conceptual frameworks within which to accommodate such phenomena.

American researcher Kendall Johnson recorded a number of striking images of the effects of zen meditation practices and acupuncture on the electrophotographic image.[21] Earle Lane has similarly recorded remarkable electrophotographic images of the effects of transcendental meditation and the use of high doses of Panax ginseng.[22] And H.S. Dakin obtained extraordinarily challenging images while working with metal-bender Uri Geller in 1973 and with psychic healer John Scudder in 1974.[23] The ideas of Rupert Sheldrake appear similarly to have been shelved until we enter a climate more favourable to the scientific investigation of the numinous and elusive.[24]

A naturopath quoted earlier identified 'the naturopathic arena' as fertile soil in which such notions can take root and find expression. Yet homoeopaths, acupuncturists and practitioners of therapeutic touch have long been cultivating similar soil. Another osteopath offers his own view of what may lie ahead:

> I foresee in my lifetime that probably the orthodoxy of the day will have some of the things that we used to think of as being radically different. As old men we might stand around saying, 'Did you see that? I don't believe it! There's a professor of medicine on the television saying the patient's aura was disrupted around the tumour.' And they might develop that. Now you already see that. If you just watch the television carefully, you are already starting to see things like that occurring.

This osteopath sees the current limits of acceptable knowledge as pushing out rapidly. A professor of medicine is a high symbol of medical authority and accomplishment. This image is used here to project what is at present an uncharted and heretical diagnostic notion, the direct vision and interpretation of the body's radiations. If such realities are truly part of the phenomenal world, they will sooner or later come to light. They are not and cannot be the exclusive domain of any one cultural or professional group. These realities will in time come to be investigated through the use of methods and technologies that perhaps have yet to be developed. Then will begin what Thomas Kuhn has termed 'the extraordinary investigations that lead the profession at last to a new set of commitments, a new basis for the practice of science'.[25]

A deepening vision

It may be helpful to revisit the ideas of Swiss philosopher Jean Gebser in the difficult quest to understand the nature of perceptions that are not universally acknowledged as real or as valid. Consciousness itself is a variable phenomenon. Although it is intangible, ungraspable and unmeasurable, our individual consciousness determines to a large extent our sense of meaning, and our capacity for understanding.

Gebser holds that humanity as a whole is presently in the process of undergoing a major mutation of consciousness characterised by what he terms 'the concretion of the spiritual'. This unusual expression reflects an attempt by Gebser to counter the notion that spirit represents an abstraction, a linguistic metaphor similar to such terms as vitality, intelligence, soul or mind. For Gebser, as for many others, the term spirit signifies not so much an extra-mundane and incorporeal presence, but denotes rather a vibrant, coherent and increasingly visible energetic presence in the world:

> The grand painful path of consciousness emergence, or, more appropriately, the unfolding and intensification of consciousness, manifests itself as an increasingly intense luminescence of spirit in man.[26]

Gebser here suggests that the current debate regarding the very existence of an energetic dimension associated with living processes may be short-lived. At present, relatively few individuals appear to be capable of perceiving and reporting upon their experiences in regard to the subtle energies associated with living systems. Perhaps this has always been the case. But one does not need to look far to realise that such perceptions have been part of human experience throughout history. Five centuries ago, Paracelsus offered the following description of what he considered to be useful attributes for any who wish to take on the mantle of healing:

> The physician should speak of that which is invisible. What is visible should belong to his knowledge, and he should recognise the illnesses just as

everybody else, who is not a physician, can recognise them by their symptoms. But this is far from making him a physician; he becomes a physician only when he knows that which is unnamed, invisible and immaterial, yet efficacious.[27]

As we know, the development of medical science has resulted in a vast knowledge of the visible, and a near-perfect understanding of the relationship between the patient's symptoms and the diseases which they signify. But a deep knowledge of the unnamed, the invisible and the immaterial has yet to be attained.

The osteopath quoted earlier draws from his own experience and from popular culture to suggest that we can no longer evade what becomes increasingly obvious for increasing numbers of people. Regardless of its origins or its nature, the so-called aura is understood to be part of spiritual reality and is available to human consciousness. According to Gebser, the perception of spiritual energies becomes more widespread as humanity moves collectively towards an intensification in consciousness. A number of respondents suggest that this phenomenon (or, more correctly, *noumenon*) will come under increasing medical scrutiny as the boundaries of the acceptable begin to broaden. Our osteopath continues:

> I don't think that everyone that's in alternative medicine is a more sensitive and loving person compared to anyone else, but they have definitely given time to develop those senses. Medicine and the healers of every tribe have always been sensitive to other things. And we know some people are sensitive to energies, some people to auras, lights, just inflections in voice, you know. You develop this, you can learn it.

The training of practitioners in many of the modalities of complementary medicine has traditionally tended to emphasise the humanistic dimensions of learning to a far greater extent than that which characterises undergraduate programs of biomedicine.

A humanistically oriented education will tend to encourage a more leisurely exploration of interior realities. This may help to sensitise practitioners to the subtler influences within life, be they related to lifestyle, relationships, emotions or spirituality. This of itself will further the development of a more holistic consciousness that will find its own expression in clinical practice. The quote above recognises sensitivity as a perennial attribute of many who aspire to the role of physician and healer. Our osteopath further raises the notion that through active training, one can consciously develop a heightened sensitivity to the subtle communications and energies that enable us to more readily participate in the life-world of others.

Such attributes need to be intrinsically valued before they can become part of the education and training of healers. The biomedical establishment remains largely sceptical of the reality of the energetic dimension that appears to be integral to many of the modalities of complementary medicine.

Between paradigms

There has always existed a strong tendency for powerful institutions to control both the thought and conduct of their members. This holds as strongly today as it did in dynastic Egypt and Renaissance Europe. Egyptian doctors were forbidden to depart from the established norms of treatment under fear of punishment. Giordano Bruno was burned alive for defending the notion that the earth moved around the sun. Galileo Galilei chose rather to bend and recanted, under threat of excommunication, his own observation that the earth truly moved around the sun. Thankfully, we live in more clement times.

Yet many who work within both medical orthodoxy and more particularly in the various modalities of complementary medicine continue to experience the opprobrium of a powerful institution, particularly if their philosophical viewpoints or treatment methods do not conform to the standards determined by the dominant system.

One of Thomas Kuhn's more valuable contributions has been his reminder that much of the scientific knowledge held as sacrosanct at any given time is in fact contingent and relative. The present form of biomedicine is itself a reflection of the philosophies, epistemologies and technologies that have developed in the Western world in recent centuries. It does not represent the omega point of the healing mission, but is more in the nature of a transient social, professional and institutional phenomenon with its own share of problems and contradictions.

The institution of biomedicine is strongly reflective of the science, philosophy and methods that have shaped it, and although immensely powerful and effective in certain areas of management and treatment, it remains but one of a number of possible approaches to the problem of human suffering borne of sickness and disease.

The growing confirmation of the influence of mind and spirit in human experience will continue to quietly push the boundaries that define the practice of contemporary scientific medicine. As attention turns towards the role of more subtle influences on our health and wellbeing through the development of new methods of research and new philosophies, the style of medicine as we know it in Western communities will inevitably change.

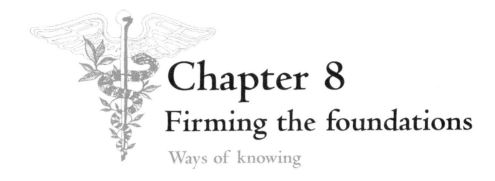

Chapter 8
Firming the foundations
Ways of knowing

A man is known better by his questions than by his answers.

Thomas Merton, 1965[1]

We need a new model of health that does not entail more medicine, more doctors, more hospitals, more drugs, or more money.

Kenneth Pelletier, 1994[2]

Historically, the practice of medicine has been bound to traditional ways and transmitted wisdom. Prior to the development of scientific method, medical knowledge represented a treasure that was painstakingly gained through familiarity with the works of ancient physicians and through constant reflection on the experiences of life. The attainment of such knowledge was understood to be one of the projects of philosophy. There was no certainty in this process; one had only the stories of those who had gone before, and the insights gained through one's own direct experiences.

Everything changed as a result of the scientific revolution. René Descartes provided the blueprint for a systematic method of gaining certain knowledge about the world. The traditional understandings of medicine were soon overtaken as the methods of science turned towards understanding the nature of the body and its diseases. Within a few short centuries, a medical revolution had occurred, and an entirely new body of knowledge that was radically different to anything that had preceded it had arisen.

Yet many of the philosophies, understandings and treatment methods that had been used since ancient times were never entirely put aside. And beyond Europe and the Western world, indigenous traditions of medicine based on differing understandings to those of the new medicine continued to be widely practised.

In recent decades, many within Western communities have begun to seek out other ways of healing and have turned to the modalities of complementary medicine. Many of those modalities are based on methods that have been used over long periods of time. The various herbal medicine traditions, for example, have been developed over millennia. And both the theory and practice of acupuncture have similarly developed over thousands of years.

The value of such approaches to healing is not dependant upon a systematic validation of their effectiveness through the methods of science. Of greater importance is the philosophical understanding of the nature of health and disease that underlies their methods. The modalities of complementary medicine represent not so much a collection of unusual therapeutic approaches but are, rather, repositories of differing perspectives on the nature of health and disease to that of biomedicine. They point to the fact that there are many ways of understanding the complexities embodied in human life.

Complementary medicine

The term 'complementary medicine' is worth reflecting upon. A complement is something that is different, yet integral, to that which it complements. Each complementary element helps support and even complete the other. Neither is fully sufficient in itself. Yet the use of the term as it relates to the therapeutic approaches other than those of biomedicine remains problematic. The relationship between biomedicine and complementary medicine is clearly not a relationship between equals or even near-equals. During the late 1980s, British sociologist Margaret Stacey conjectured on how both the dominant biomedicine and the ascendant non-orthodox modalities would deal with each other's influence:

> It certainly seems likely that biomedicine will seek to co-opt the more popular of alternative healing modes, making them subservient to biomedically trained practitioners. Those modes would then be called 'complementary', not 'alternative'. How strongly will alternative healers resist becoming complements (handmaidens?) of biomedicine? Or will they be so anxious for recognition that they will propose such an answer themselves?[3]

Perhaps Stacey's ascription of handmaiden status to complementary medicine may have been too harsh a judgement. Regardless, in the intervening time, the term complementary has become both fully established and fully acceptable to all parties. The subordinate position of complementary medicine, however, continues to be evidenced in the demands made by biomedicine for validation of efficacy of its therapeutic approaches.

Despite the differing character of diagnostic modes and treatment methods, there remains strong pressure that the modalities of complementary medicine be assessed according to criteria developed primarily for the testing of pharmaceutical drugs on specific diseases or conditions. Yet there are strong arguments that the more holistic styles of complementary medicine require the use of research methods that more appropriately reflect the differing styles of both diagnosis and treatment used in the various modalities.

At a technical level, biomedicine is without peer historically and culturally. Yet a number of problems have been identified at other levels. The clinical style of most Western physicians has been strongly conditioned by their scientific training and many years of internship in hospital environments. This may limit the degree of expression of the doctor as artist, skilfully able to read the subtle verbal and behavioural clues that may point in unexpected directions.

In addition, the uniformity of treatment methods leaves little room for the exploration of non-orthodox ways to address issues in patients' lives that may have a bearing either on their disposition to illness, or their strength of recovery. More autonomously inclined patients may be more interested in knowing what they can do for themselves than what can be done for them. And both doctors and patients have begun to ask whether there may be other approaches than exclusively drug-based solutions to the problems associated with ageing and chronic disease. Attention has begun to turn more strongly towards preventative measures, and towards methods that focus more on the enhancement of health than on the controlling of disease symptoms through the use of powerful drugs.

The modalities of complementary medicine have provided a useful lens to identify some of those shortfalls and a mirror to reflect differing perspectives that may, in time, help restore balance to the healing project. They offer other approaches to both diagnosis and treatment, and add significantly to the options available to a public already well served at every stage in life by the methods of biomedicine.

Having gained in cultural acceptability in recent years, the modalities of complementary medicine are now called upon to justify their credentials, and to show through systematic testing that they are indeed effective and do in fact hold significant healing potential for patients. The question, of course, is how this is to be realised to everybody's satisfaction.

A call for evidence, or the burden of proof?

Biomedicine has long cleaved to the view that scientific method is the best way of gaining knowledge about the body and its workings. That knowledge has proven its usefulness repeatedly over the past century. The power of that knowledge has been reinforced by the influence of the many institutions associated with medical education and research. In addition, the widespread utilisation of proven medical technologies and the ubiquitous presence of powerful drug companies ensure that the present models of biomedical investigation and treatment will continue to be favoured over other approaches.

The institutional power of complementary medicine, on the other hand, has been until recently virtually non-existent. Training colleges tended to be privately owned, tuition fees were drawn directly from students without government support or assistance, texted sources were few and often rudimentary and research culture had yet to develop in any meaningful way. This situation has begun to change in recent years. The movement of complementary medicine education into university environments has provided unprecedented access to library resources, technical facilities, an established research culture and government funding.

The rise of complementary medicine has come about as a direct result of popular support and by the exercise of choice on the part of numerous individual patients. An osteopath reflects:

The orthodox, begrudgingly, is moving towards what the public is demanding—not towards us necessarily—but towards what the public is demanding. That is, more time, more sensitivity and more general family practice. Not necessarily the high-tech stuff.

Despite the absence of formal proof of efficacy, stories of benefits received by patients have been told in so many quarters that many practitioners of biomedicine have adopted a guarded empiricism and are beginning to test for themselves the truth of their patients' reports of the helpfulness of other approaches to healing.

The randomised controlled trial

The science of clinical validation has been brought to its highest pitch through the randomised controlled trial (RCT). This method of clinical evaluation was formally incorporated into the methods of biomedicine in the 1940s. It represents the ultimate standard for determining with certainty whether a specific medical intervention alters the natural progression of a given condition or disease entity. Medical philosopher Edmund Pellegrino spells out the role of the RCT in the practice of biomedicine:

> What distinguishes modern therapeutics is not its superior rationality, but its scientific epistemology. Effectiveness is judged by the tests of scientific evidence, not by conformity to an all-encompassing theory, the details of a preset ritual, or the exhib-ition of some physiological response like emesis, diuresis, or catharsis. Effectiveness in modern therapeutics is defined as the capability of an agent, demonstrably and measurably, to alter the statistically predictable natural history of the disease.[4]

Built into the randomised controlled trial are controls to ensure that those tested are representative of the general population, and controls for experimenter bias that may influence the outcome of a given study. Further controls may be introduced to counter the influence of non-specific or placebo-type effects. Research findings are analysed using statistical procedures to determine whether a given therapeutic intervention has a greater-than-chance influence upon the natural progression of the disease-entity or symptom-group under investigation.

There can be no question that such methods are supremely appropriate to the biomedical epistemology, based as it is on reductionist foundations. Randomised clinical trials were developed primarily to evaluate the safety and efficacy of a specific clinical intervention, usually the administration of a newly synthesised drug, on a specific clinical entity.

The attempt to impose such standards upon complementary medicine treatments is fraught with difficulty. Firstly, the diagnostic categories used to describe pathology or disharmony will often differ significantly from those of biomedicine. Traditonal Chinese medicine educator Manfred Porkert offers both clarity and insight regarding some of the differences between the diagnostic methods of traditional Chinese medicine and those of biomedicine:

> The analytic and causal methodology of Western medicine calls for active intervention in order to identify precisely the antecedent causes of the observed symptoms and the somatic substratum involved. The Chinese physician, in contrast, is interested in the present functions and actual symptoms of the patient. *Szu-chen*—his four diagnostic methods: inspection, interrogation, auscultation/olfaction, and palpation of the six radial pulses—are all aimed at a complete appraisal of the momentary functional situation of the patient. The data he looks for are directly open to the senses. Therefore the Chinese diagnostician's job consists of the rational assessment of symptoms by applying the inductive method and its qualitative standards. The fact apparently so difficult to grasp is that because of

their epistemological complementarity, Chinese and Western medicines, without one being basically inferior to the other, cannot and do not produce mutually identical results.[5]

In a similar way, homoeopathic physicians will look for patterns in the totality of the patient's presentation rather than for identifiable pathologies within specific organ systems. This is not to say that biomedical diagnoses are not relevant to such approaches. But the overall assessment and management of patients will be determined largely by such qualitative considerations.

Secondly, complementary approaches often involve the use of multiple interventions, formulated on an individual basis, in the treatment of patients. A naturopath may therefore prescribe a herbal formulation, which itself may be made up of a number of individual medicinal plants, mineral supplementation, a high potency constitutional homoeopathic medicine, spinal adjustment and dietary modification as integral parts of the treatment program. In addition, suggestions may also be offered in regard to patterns of work and activity and to issues relating to the interior life of the patient.

Thirdly, complementary medicine interventions are rarely fixed, but will tend to vary according to how the patients' symptoms change from visit to visit. An osteopath may therefore reassess the patient structurally at each visit, and treat the patient differently as the pattern of segmental restrictions changes during recovery.

The value and the appropriateness of the RCT in the testing of certain *specific* therapeutic substances used in the treatment of *specific* conditions or disorders by practitioners of complementary medicine are beyond question. This is reflected in the scientific validation of the influence of such herbal agents as *Echinacea* on immune function, of *Ginkgo* on cerebral circulation, of *Panax ginseng* on adaptogenic capacity, of *Silybum*, or milk thistle, on liver function, and of *Serenoa*, or saw palmetto, extracts in prostatic hypertrophy.[6] But the randomised clinical trial remains of limited value in assessing the usefulness of the multivariate interventions that tend to characterise the more holistic approach of complementary medicine.

In regard to the testing of individual herbal medicines, there are further complexities that may need to be addressed. Medicinal plants may carry a single name, but they often carry many classes of active constituents, each of which may influence the overall therapeutic effect. A single plant extract, therefore, may contain minerals, flavonoids, volatile oils, polyphenols and steroidal compounds, each of which may carry subtle healing influences. A practitioner of herbal medicine reflects:

The medicine in itself is powerful, and as more research is done, the picture becomes clearer as to why the medicines are powerful:

flavonoids across the board, the enormous properties of flavonoids; the tannins, which were not taken seriously up until five years ago; and now mucilage, which was always regarded as a waste product, now showing immuno-modulating properties. And I think as they research it more, and have an understanding of the chemistry, that helps to explain it combined with the practitioner–patient interaction, and just this holistic approach to it.

The constellation of influences that operate within even a single plant medicine will often vary according to such factors as climatic conditions, soil type and time of harvest. Each of these factors may influence the balance of constituents produced within any given plant. Because of the need for specificity and reproducibility in scientific research, such problematic issues have been 'overcome' by manipulating the levels of one or another of the active constituents of plants in order to approximate a standard replicable extract, as has occurred in the testing of *Echinacea, Hypericum* and *Ginkgo*. But there are many within the herbal medicine community who would argue that such solutions are not consistent with the holistic basis of their approach.

Beyond such polemics, the contemporary clinical testing of pharmaceutical drugs is very expensive. Huge amounts of money are needed to bring even a single new drug into the medical marketplace. Richard Smith, editor of the *British Medical Journal*, has recently noted:

Drug companies spend hundred of millions of pounds to bring a new drug to market, and tens of millions of pounds to do the clinical trials that are necessary for both registration and marketing.[7]

Apart from issues relating to the appropriateness of such methodologies in the testing of complementary medicine, the sheer cost of the project could simply not be sustained at the present time. The resources and infrastructure needed to conduct clinical trials have been created by the biomedical establishment over the course of the past century. Drug development, testing, manufacture and marketing are major operations conducted by drug companies whose global operations and economic resources are on a similar scale to those of multinational oil companies.

In 1997, the National Institute of Health in the United States funded a study to test the efficacy of *Hypericum perforatum* (St John's wort) in the treatment of clinical depression. The amount allocated for the trial, which involved 300 patients, was US$4.5 million.[8] And this was a single trial of a single medicinally active plant. It is worth keeping in mind that over 240 individual medicinal plants have been listed and described in the three volumes of the *British Herbal Pharmacopeia*. And over 320 medicinal plants are represented in the Commission E monographs developed for practitioners of herbal medicine in the European community.[9] Many hundreds of medicinally active plants are also used in each of the materia medica of the Ayurvedic and traditional Chinese systems of medicine.

A major element of the present impasse lies in the attempt to assess holistic systems of medicine using reductionist research methods. As we have seen, this can be done in a limited way with a small number of therapeutic substances. But behind such programs, there is probably lurking a hefty business plan built on the possibility of the global marketing of a patentable, standardised extract that can be prescribed in the manner of existing pharmaceuticals. A naturopath cynically comments:

> There is a danger within our own realm that we just become alternative medical prescribers, being more rigid, being more fundamentalist, and being perhaps in some senses, more blinkered. So what you have now . . . is the therapist who's going to fix it all. 'You've got a headache? We've got a headache herb combo.' And so we are getting in a sense our own pharmaceutical industry.

What is more urgently needed than the validation of individual plant medicines or individual therapeutic procedures for specific conditions is the development of research methods capable of assessing holistic approaches that offer multidimensional solutions to what are often multidimensional problems.

Finding new ways

At its present stage of development, complementary medicine remains poorly described. Before its particular styles of intervention or individual treatment approaches can be usefully subjected to the degree of scrutiny demanded by the biomedical model of assessment of efficacy, there is much work to be done in simply identifying the essential character of complementary medicine.

The holism that finds expression in the modalities of complementary medicine carries both diagnostic styles and treatment methods that differ markedly from those of biomedicine. In addition, the foundational elements of complementary medicine incorporate concepts that at present remain questionable for many within biomedicine. These include such notions as the healing potential of the relationship between physician and patient, the activation of inherent healing capacities within the patient, the role of mind and spirit in the healing process, the multi-causal origins of many diseases and much ill-health within the community, and the value of multidimensional rather than specific interventions in the treatment of disease and the restoration of health.

Unlike biomedicine, complementary medicine does not represent a unified or codified system of healing, even though a number of its modalities are based upon integral philosophical understandings. Complementary medicine carries a variety of different therapeutic styles that range from the physical to the energetic, from the use of therapeutic substances to the implementation of dietary change, from the encouragement of exercise programs to instruction in relaxation or guided visualisation.

The calls for the implementation of research programs capable of assessing the diverse interventions that characterise holistic approaches to treatment represent but one pole in the work of validating the potential contribution of complementary medicine to health care. There is an equally pressing need for descriptive studies that can provide needed insight into the meaning and influence of such interventions in the lives of both practitioners and patients. What do patients themselves have to say about their experiences with complementary medicine? Why do they choose such therapies over more orthodox approaches? How do those who practise complementary medicine see themselves in relation to practitioners of biomedicine?

Studies designed to address such questions do not need the huge resources necessary to test individual interventions or treatments to the satisfaction of established models of biomedical research. They can be readily carried out using the networks and supports made newly available by the entry of complementary medicine into university environments.

Well-conducted interpretive research can provide useful information regarding the motivation and experiences of both practitioners and patients of complementary medicine. It can similarly provide an early mapping of the more experiential domains of healing. Such research may better enable an identification of those conditions for which complementary medicine offers greater benefits than the methods of biomedicine. Such studies may open up many valuable leads for more specific clinical investigations.

At another level, interpretive or qualitative studies may reflect back to biomedicine the way that it is perceived by both the general community and by health care practitioners who operate outside of the biomedical framework. This may help bring back into focus the hidden assumptions of biomedicine that are often masked by too strong an emphasis upon quantitative determinations of the effectiveness of therapeutic interventions.[10]

Descriptive studies can more easily focus upon the role of such elusive elements as lifestyle, personal motivation and the role of the doctor–patient relationship in the healing process. These are tenuous issues that are not easily formulated or simply resolved. Such studies can provide a broader platform from which an integrated approach to health care based more upon holistic than reductionistic principles may be developed.

Health in the suburbs

During the 1980s, North American sociologist Meredith McGuire and her colleagues undertook a major study addressing these more subtle dimensions of healing. *Ritual Healing in Suburban America* details the results of a wide-ranging qualitative investigation of both practitioners and clients of 'non-medical' healing methods. The study was based on a series of depth interviews and participant observation of over 130 different groups of non-orthodox healers, healing groups and patients. Participants in the study included practitioners of psychic healing, Christian healing and yoga, as well as practitioners of the more conventional complementary modalities of chiropractic, naturopathy, homoeopathy and acupuncture.

McGuire's study confirmed the common human desire for autonomy in matters of health. Self-medication has traditionally been the first line of approach to the problem of sickness throughout history. Despite the impressive structures developed around the institution of medicine and the cultural power exercised by practitioners of biomedicine, self-medication and the desire for freedom from overarching control continue to determine the choices that many make in relation to their own health and that of their families. As McGuire states:

> These data show that even the strangest, most difficult to understand healing beliefs and practices provide very important functions for their adherents: meaning, order and a sense of personal empowerment in the face of upsetting or even traumatic experiences in life. Alternative healing systems are meeting some people's needs, which the dominant system does not address. Thus they highlight some of the limits of modern 'scientific' medicine.[11]

Meredith McGuire and her colleagues draw attention to a number of issues that have, by and large, been discounted or dismissed in the dominant model of Western medicine. These issues figure prominently in the lives of many who choose to use non-orthodox methods of healing. This study draws attention to the symbolic dimension of illness and identifies this as an active element in the life-world of many who work outside of the dominant paradigm. It also points towards the essential failure of biomedicine to adequately address the social, economic and cultural realities that presently contribute to the pandemic of chronic disease engulfing an otherwise burgeoning Western civilisation.

Those interviewed in this study represented 'middle-class, middle-aged, well educated, socially, culturally and residentially established suburbanites'.[12]

McGuire's research suggests that those who make use of non-orthodox approaches do so in order to better understand and manage their own sicknesses and in order to participate more fully in the processes that lead to a restoration of their health:

> These respondents are asserting an alternative model of medical practice—one in which the patient exerts greater power and control. They seek a different quality of doctor–patient communication—a model in which doctors serve as knowledgeable resource persons for self-aware patients. Such communication would, accordingly, consist of much information exchange and mutual respect. It would also be (in the ideal image of respondents) open to non-medical alternatives, which patients could choose as respectable options in their health-seeking.[13]

Descriptive studies such as that undertaken by McGuire and her colleagues are categorically different from the randomised clinical trials that have become identified with valid medical research. They cannot determine with certainty the usefulness or otherwise of specific therapeutic interventions. But what they do provide are powerful methods for identifying structural issues within the medical project that may influence the experiences of patients for better or worse. Such studies enable the identification of blind spots within clinical reality that have been overlooked in the day-to-day practise of medicine. The methods of qualitative research can provide a needed corrective to an approach to medical research that has for much of the past century focused more upon the disease and its treatment than upon the person and their experience of sickness or ill-health.

Meredith McGuire has explored the experiential dimensions of health and sickness. The view offered in her important study is deserving of a broader audience than a small group of academic sociologists.

Health in the corporate world

During the 1990s, Kenneth Pelletier and his colleagues at Stanford University School of Medicine undertook a major study also using qualitative research methods. Rather than focusing upon practitioners of non-orthodox medicine or their patrons, Pelletier and his colleagues looked at the health practices of an elite group within American society. His *Sound Mind, Sound Body: A new model for lifelong health* represents a descriptive study based on depth interviews with '53 prominent individuals who represent prototypes of optimal health'.[14]

Although the notion of optimal health is open to interpretation, Pelletier selected his respondents on the basis of their accomplishments as acknowledged by their professional and business peers, on their adherence to personal health practices and on their commitment to ethical and spiritual values. Pelletier's study offers considerable insight into those personal choices that enable certain individuals to maintain high levels of personal health, creativity and productivity throughout their lives. His research revealed that such qualities as personal courage and the capacity for perseverance in the face of difficulties may be of more importance in the maintenance of health and the overcoming of health problems than any amount of medication or supplementation.

In focusing upon health rather than disease, Pelletier effectively overturned the traditional biomedical perspective. In the process, he too confirmed the centrality of personal autonomy in both health creation and health maintenance. Those interviewed valued highly their own independence and freedom of choice, and generally sought out whatever therapeutic approaches they found to be helpful, regardless of whether or not they were sanctioned by orthodox medicine, in order to deal with their occasional sicknesses:

> The majority of participants regularly sought out such treatments as acupuncture, massage and therapeutic touch, homoeopathy, herbal remedies, chiropractic, macrobiotics, and most frequently, mind–body practices, including hypnosis, biofeedback and meditation.[15]

Like McGuire, Pelletier was not dealing with a group of disaffected fringe-dwellers seeking out alternatives to the mainstream. His respondents were high flyers within US corporate culture and professional life. Their choices are a silent yet powerful indictment of the inability of biomedicine to respond to the *health* needs of many within the community. These findings reflect a widespread knowledge that there are more ways to restore health than drugs and surgery.

Pelletier's work was carried out in his role as Director of Stanford's Corporate Health Program. It was largely driven by the needs of American corporate capitalism rather than by the support of government agencies or the profession of medicine itself.

Ironically, programs such as those developed by Pelletier and his colleagues may prove to be more influential in benefiting the health of many within American society than the promotional activities of government-based health education departments.

The principles uncovered by Pelletier and his colleagues have major implications for the way that community medicine can be practised.

The bridge builders

More recently, Bruce Barrett and his colleagues from the University of Wisconsin Medical School surveyed practitioners of complementary medicine in their immediate neighbourhood in order to better understand how such practitioners view themselves and their biomedical colleagues.

> We were particularly interested in exploring CAM (complementary and alternative medicine) practitioners' ideas regarding the possibilities of integrating conventional, complementary and alternative perspectives, practices and systems.[16]

Barrett's study was based on depth interviews with 32 individual practitioners. As well as including representatives of such modalities as traditional Chinese medicine, chiropractic, herbalism, homoeopathy and naturopathy, respondents also included practitioners of colonic irrigation, Feldenkreis, Rolfing, tai ch'i, yoga and astrology. This eclectic spread reflects the broader range of non-orthodox healing modalities encompassed by the term 'complementary and alternative' which is commonly used in North America.

A number of important findings emerged from the study. Those interviewed identified their primary work as the treatment of chronic, rather than acute, conditions. Many of their patients had already been through the treadmill of conventional biomedical treatments with little apparent benefit. Barrett's respondents viewed themselves not only as healers and facilitators of healing processes but, more importantly, as educators. They identified their approach as being essentially holistic. They attributed a large part of their effectiveness to the fact that they were able to get to know and understand their clients better through the freedom offered by unhurried consultations. They accepted that a major part of their task centred on empowerment of their clients by the encouragement of autonomy and self-reliance in health matters.

Those interviewed generally understood their work to be complementary rather than antagonistic to that of biomedicine. Their individualised approach helped patients to gain a deeper understanding of their health problems through becoming more informed and more reflective. All respondents welcomed the prospect of closer interaction with their biomedical colleagues. They were far more interested in serving the needs of their patients than in protecting their own occupational territory, or justifying their freedom to practise.

Like the earlier studies of McGuire and Pelletier, Barrett's work strongly supports the notion that individual health is better served through the incorporation into health care of the holistic principles utilised by many practitioners of complementary medicine. The continuing problem, of course, remains how best to determine the nature and the extent of the benefits.

Wisdom from the desert

Regardless of whether the methods of complementary medicine have been formally validated or not, it has by now become clear that they are perceived by both practitioners and patients as fulfilling certain needs that are not fulfilled by more conventional approaches. In addition, many who choose to make use of those methods report that they enjoy significant health benefits.

The University of Arizona College of Medicine has, since 1975, incorporated elements of complementary medicine into its undergraduate medical program.[17] It was among the first within biomedicine to correctly identify the nature of the challenge presented by the increasing use of complementary medicine throughout the Western world.

The rise of complementary medicine called attention to a number of structural deficiencies within the biomedical approach to health and disease. It added significantly to the momentum that shifted biomedicine towards an expansion of its conceptual understanding of the nature of health and disease, and a broadening of the range of 'acceptable' therapeutic approaches. It hastened a deepening realisation that medicine is as much an art as a science, that health resides as much in harmony as in biochemistry, and that the mystery of healing transcends procedure and technique.

In a beautifully crafted review of the changing status of contemporary biomedicine and the need for changes in the way medical research is conducted, Iris Bell and her colleagues at the University of Arizona have suggested a number of ways in which current research methods can be extended in order to more accurately serve the needs of a medicine in process of transition from a biologically oriented reductionist paradigm to an holistic systems-oriented integrative paradigm:

> The nature of medical research itself can and must expand beyond the prevailing reductionist approaches and quantitative study designs to measure the systemic effectiveness of integrative medical practice.[18]

Like Bruce Barrett and his colleagues from the Wisconsin School of Medicine, Iris Bell and her colleagues take an essentially meliorist stance towards the non-biomedical healing modalities, and appear to sit comfortably with their differing philosophical foundations and clinical practises. They accept that diseases often result from multiple rather than single causes;

that desirable and valid outcomes for therapeutic interventions should include psychological, social and spiritual as well as biological dimensions of patients' lives; and that treatments or therapeutic programs may require multiple rather than single interventions.

The RCT has, for many decades, resolved all uncertainties regarding the efficacy or otherwise of biomedical interventions. It is supremely appropriate for testing the effects of singular substances or single interventions upon specified disease processes in a representative population. But the rules of the game begin to change. The biochemical model upon which most drug testing was based has extended to a broader systems approach that includes the role of psychological, social, environmental and spiritual influences.

The Arizona group has called for the use of broad-based observational studies to provide an early mapping of the effectiveness of the often complex interventions that characterise holistic approaches to medicine. They are not alone in that suggestion.[19] Observational studies offer a valuable and more formal complement to the weight of historical evidence supporting the use of treatment methods such as traditional Chinese medicine, Ayurveda and the various systems of herbal medicine. Although these ancient systems have not been formally validated by the methods of science, they have been empirically tested by generations of healers, and by centuries of experience.

A practitioner of Western herbal medicine reminds us that biomedicine has perhaps too hastily dismissed many of the traditions from which it has itself emerged:

> The difference is they [patients] are getting better. Their pain is subsiding, their quality of life is improving, their skin condition is getting better, the child's asthma is getting better, their periods are stabilising. They're getting better. Why are they getting better? Well, herbal medicine has a long tradition, a long tradition. And the reality is that if that medicine had not performed over the centuries, it would not have lasted. Full stop. It's as basic as that.

Iris Bell and her colleagues have urged that medical researchers become more familiar with the qualitative research models developed by sociologists and behavioural scientists to study the complex multivariate dimensions that characterise social reality. Such skills may prove useful in the work ahead.

It will take some time yet before there is a more general acceptance of the appropriateness and usefulness of these newer methods of evaluation. The present discourse reflects a deepening awareness that research methods will need to accommodate both the multi-causal understanding of disease causation and the multi-intervention treatment strategies that characterise more holistic approaches. As Thomas Kuhn has noted:

Normal science can proceed without rules so long as the relevant scientific community accepts without question the particular problem-solutions already achieved. Rules should therefore become important and the characteristic unconcern about them should vanish whenever paradigms or models are felt to be insecure. That is, moreover, exactly what does occur. The pre-paradigm period, in particular, is regularly marked by frequent and deep debates over legitimate methods, problems and standards of solution, though these serve rather to define schools than to produce agreement.[20]

The determination of the effectiveness of new or unfamiliar treatment programs is a necessary part of *scientia*, the knowledge that leads to discernment and enables decisions to be based upon truth rather than conjecture. The acquisition of that knowledge in relation to the treatment methods of complementary medicine will require a sustained commitment to the incorporation of holistic principles into the research methods themselves.

The changing rules

The pain, limitation and physical incapacitation that are often associated with sickness and disease belong to the patient. Regardless of whether a given drug has been proven many times over by placebo-controlled clinical trials, if a patient continues to experience distress, if comfort is compromised, or if the side effects of prescribed drugs are found to be too disturbing, the decision may be taken to look elsewhere with or without the approval of the family doctor. The increasing cultural acceptance and ready availability of practitioners of complementary medicine have made it easier to find out for oneself whether there are better ways of dealing with those health problems for which conventional biomedical approaches can provide only limited relief or benefit.

Individual patients will form their own judgements on the basis of their own experience. A mother will become understandably frustrated when her child is prescribed a fourth successive course of antibiotics during a given winter. The development of stomach pain after using anti-inflammatory medication for low back pain may prompt one to visit a chiropractor or osteopath, or to swim in the local pool a little more often. The decision to seek out other ways of dealing with difficult or recurrent symptoms may lead not only to deepened insight into the nature of those symptoms, but to unexpected benefits beyond the immediate condition. A homoeopath reflects:

Often people have been to four or five different practitioners and they might find that one or two are much more helpful for them. That to me is a form of empowerment because they know who to go to for what. They also learn, say with acute episodes of problems, what medicines to take by themselves. And they also learn about diet and so on. I mean, the ideal is to make them much more aware of what is good for their bodies and what's good for their psyche.

This comment alludes to an attitude on the part of the patient that will actively seek a resolution to their symptoms and the restoration of their health. The autonomously inclined will not be content to pursue a course of treatment that provides palliation without resolution. They will tend to look further. They may well try out a number of different approaches in order to best determine, for themselves, where the benefit lies. In the process, they may learn more of 'what is good for their bodies and what's good for their psyche' from their homoeopath than from their medical practitioner.

The movement of patients to the modalities of complementary medicine grew steadily throughout the Western world over the last three decades of the twentieth century. It is now widely understood, both by practitioners and by patients generally, that despite its awesome power in such domains as emergency medicine and surgery, and despite its deep knowledge of the body and its diseases, scientific medicine represents only one of a number of possible ways of dealing with health problems. This understanding has clearly penetrated the ranks of the medical profession, and is reflected in the incorporation of elements of complementary medicine education in the curricula of many medical schools in the United States, Europe and Australia.[21]

There appears to be a growing acceptance by many within medicine of the need to become more familiar not only with the methods of complementary medicine, but with those who practise them with competence and understanding. The issue is no longer a political one. It rests, as it has always ultimately rested, on the health and wellbeing of patients. A naturopath comments:

It's the successes of what we've been able to demonstrate clinically that has been observed by enough doctors over a long period of time now, that they are actually slowly starting to turn around and at least honour that we may have some value to offer. So as that is seen more and more, doctors will change their practice.

This has certainly come to pass. This reflection from a practitioner of naturopathic medicine carries the essential meaning of the phenomenon of complementary medicine. The modalities of complementary medicine represent far more than mere repositories of unusual and archaic techniques of healing which should be tested according to the rules of biomedicine. Their significance lies not so much in the details, but rather in the philosophies on which they are based, and on the understanding of health and sickness carried in their methods.

The confirmation by placebo-controlled clinical trials that *Ginkgo biloba* extracts improve cerebral circulation and are effective in the treatment of certain forms of tinnitus and vertigo is certainly welcome news. And it is similarly satisfying to learn the details, uncovered through elegant experimental work, of the mechanisms whereby the pharmacologically active constituents of *Ginkgo* exert their influence. But what is more important, and more influential in the longer term, is a recovery of the knowledge of the principles underlying those systems of healing from which such medicines as *Ginkgo* are derived.

Outer intervention or inner motivation?

The call for validation of holistic approaches to healing has brought about a re-evaluation of the essential meaning and utility of non-specific, or placebo-type, effects in healing.[22] Within the reductionist paradigm of biomedical research, placebo effects represent a nuisance that can interfere with the certain determination of whether a specific drug or procedure is capable of altering the natural history of a specific diagnostic entity. Such considerations are of crucial importance in the testing of newly synthesised drugs that have never been used before as medicines. But from another perspective, all means that lead to an improvement in the state of the patient are to be welcomed, regardless of whether they originate in the alteration of the biochemistry of the body, from a change in the pattern of activities in a person's life, or from a change in mental attitude.

In addition, from the holistic perspective, the issue of what actually facilitates the change in the patient is not crucial. The change itself is the key consideration. That change may come through the agency of a synthesised drug, through a homoeopathic remedy, through osteopathic realignment, through the encouragement and support of the healer, or through a combination of any or all of these influences.

The quest for certainty in outcomes has led to a devaluation of nuance, of probability, of subtlety, of the reality of uncertainty in *any* healing endeavour. Even well-proved drugs occasionally do not work. And beyond a certain point, particularly where a person may be subject to multiple pathologies or where a chronic disease is close to having run its course, there may be very little that can be offered in the way of medication or treatment. But one's usefulness as a physician does not thereby cease.

Nothing is fixed in life, and a willingness to live with uncertainty is perhaps a necessary aspect of thoughtful practice. Sometimes the apparently simple defies all attempts at resolution. And other times, the apparently hopeless surprisingly turns for the better. A practitioner of traditional Chinese medicine reflects on such considerations:

> *I don't know whether or not the energy we manipulate is something that's sort of one with the universe, that's Godly. I mean I really don't know. I just know that I have witnessed incredible things in some people. But in other people I've really wanted to see something happen and I don't know whether it's been my poor selection of [acupuncture] points or whether or not there's been a basic blockage or something. I really don't understand. I've truly witnessed miracles and yet in other people I haven't been able to shift anything. I wish I could give you a better answer.*

The essential mystery of healing is honestly and simply expressed here. The world view of this acupuncturist clearly transcends materiality and rationality. She appears to be totally comfortable with the notion that a more-than-human intelligence may be implicated in the processes that are activated in healing. She is not concerned by the political or academic correctness of her position, and remains in awe of the mystery of the healing process to which she is daily witness. Rational justifications and explanations of how her treatments do their work remain secondary to the fact that, from her own perspective and experience, she knows the treatments to be effective, sometimes remarkably so.

The call for validation of the methods of complementary medicine cannot be satisfied by the systematic subjection of individual treatments or individual medicines to costly, time-consuming and logistically difficult testing programs. Apart from the Gargantuan nature of such a project, it misses the essential contribution of complementary medicine to medical understanding. More of the same will do little to broaden and deepen the conceptual basis of scientific medicine.

The modalities of complementary medicine have served the important purpose of reawakening the mind of Western medicine to the holistic basis of life, to the fact that our material or bodily natures are but part of the totality within which we live. The essential task ahead calls for a sensitive integration of that understanding into the testing methods of medicine generally, and an increasing utilisation of methods of investigation that are capable of holistically assessing the outcomes of holistically based treatments.

As the understanding of medicine begins to extend beyond the materialist and reductionist principles that have carried it so far over the course of the past century, its ways of knowing will progressively reflect that transformation.

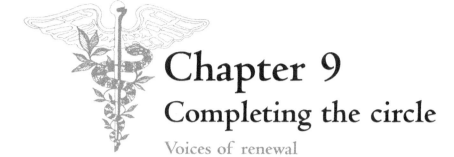

Chapter 9
Completing the circle
Voices of renewal

For all its technological power, medicine is not a technological enterprise. The practice of medicine is a special kind of love.

Rachel Naomi Remen, 1996[1]

It should be especially clear in medicine that we cannot have well humans on a sick planet. Medicine must first turn its attention to protecting the health and wellbeing of the Earth before there can be any effective human health.

Thomas Berry, 1991[2]

During the closing decades of the twentieth century, the profession of medicine in the West began to reacquire many of the holistic principles that have governed the practice of thoughtful and evolved physicianship through the ages. Ironically, this happened at a time when scientific medicine was at its most powerful, when the nature of the body and the diseases to which it is subject had been charted virtually down to the last detail, when the search for knowledge of the processes that sustain life itself had reached deeply into the creative core of cellular DNA.

With most diseases now documented and well understood, it is tempting to ask where the further movement of medicine is likely to proceed. New frontiers begin to open up in such areas as molecular genetics and embryonic research. It is as though the notion of limitless growth has seized the imagination of those on the far edge of medical research, even though such notions are ultimately unsustainable.

Although the accomplishments of biomedicine over the past century have been truly staggering, there are aspects of human suffering that call for more than technical solutions. Those living under the shadow of chronic degenerative diseases, or the so-called 'diseases of civilisation', know that they can only be propped up for so long with more drugs and more procedures.

In this time of universal knowledge and education, we need to inquire further regarding the true limits of medicine, the degree to which it is prepared to work towards healing all aspects of life as far as it is possible to do so. Is it enough to expect of medicine only that of which it is technically capable? By focusing primarily on disease, has biomedicine neglected many of the other dimensions of contemporary life that contribute to ill-health? Is the task of medicine confined to the health of the individual, or is there a duty of care towards the health of families, of communities, of the ecosystems within which we participate, and of the earth itself?

Holism inherently calls for broader perspectives. It calls for the development of an ecological sensitivity that discerns patterns of influence and interaction that extend beyond individual biology. Holistic approaches to health require both a willingness to look beyond the obvious, and an acceptance that uncertainty is part of the cost of transcending the fixed boundaries of individual pathology. An early critic of the holistic health movement in the United States has taken up this dialectic:

> Holists claim that medicine (a term that in this section will denote all conventional health-care disciplines) defines its practice too narrowly, an approach that results in dehumanising treatment of patients. Medicine is accused of focusing on the disease, the part, the technique—all at the expense, of course, of the 'whole person'. It is too much concerned, accuse the holists, with the therapy and too little with the patient. The scientific method is felt to impose too small a focus.
>
> Conventional providers, on the other hand, protest that the holists are acting irresponsibly by trying to assign every human problem to the province of health care, thereby increasing the already heavy burden of practitioners. They believe that use of the scientific method allows them to do what they do best—heal the sick—and that holism may be encouraging them to do many things badly.[3]

There are no ready answers to such questions. The issues are, by their very nature, complex. But the movement of medicine in recent decades has been more towards, rather than away from, a deepening appreciation of the nature of holism and of its role in the mission of healing. It is not that holism encourages healers to do many things badly. Holism, in fact, encourages healers to do many things well.

Simpler times

It remains a curious anomaly that scientific medicine's deep knowledge of disease and its treatment has not been matched by a similar knowledge of health and of ways that it can be maintained or augmented. That project was, perhaps, the necessity of earlier times, of times when diseases were as yet poorly understood, of times when knowledge of medicines was rudimentary.

Ancient healers sought to actively support the forces that sustained the health of their people rather than contending in often fruitless battles with diseases of which they knew little with medicines of which they knew less. In such times, effectiveness rested largely in the person of the healer, in their capacity to awaken hope in their patients, and in their ability to offer meaningful explanations of sickness that restored some order to their patients' worlds.

The priest-doctors of ancient Egypt clearly understood the importance of preventive medicine. They encouraged the use of hygienic practices to preserve the health of their people. During the time of the later dynasties, the people of the Nile delta regularly undertook a ritual cleansing of their bodies through the use of purgatives, enemas and dietary restriction. Egyptian medical historian Paul Ghalioungui recalls:

> Even the Greeks thought excessive the care that Egyptians took of their bodies. All their travellers talk with admiration of the Egyptian customs of washing the hands and the crockery, and of taking purgatives and emetics every month. These customs were certainly in large part due to the example and teaching of the priests, who practiced an extremely fastidious ritual of cleanliness and of whom Herodotus wrote that they must certainly have received many benefits to submit to these innumerable observances.[4]

Such practices, at the very least, enabled the population as a whole to better cope with the many waterborne diseases and parasites carried by the yearly flooding of their rivers and waterways. In addition, they would have conferred the benefits of metabolic renewal brought about by short periods of fasting and cleansing.

During the pre-Hippocratic period in Greece, Asklepiad physicians attended their patients both directly and through the 300 healing temples scattered throughout their land. These places of healing were generally located away from the towns and cities and provided a place of rest and renewal for those in need. Patients would bathe in the waters of the springs alongside which many of the temples were situated, and then be massaged with fragrant oils and nourished with pure foods. Periods spent in these early hospitals were times of ritual purification of the body and mind, and offered the opportunity for inner reflection and bodily recovery. The gently restorative treatments received by patients served to strengthen them during their time of recuperation.

In the present day, such systems as Indian Ayurvedic medicine and traditional Chinese medicine continue to make use of special treatments that aim primarily to strengthen and restore the physical and mental reserves of patients. These Eastern systems of medicine provide both curative treatments and time-tested methods that serve to actively increase health and vigour. Such methods include dietary regulation, yoga and tai ch'i practices, and the use of tonic plants such as ginseng, or the restorative *rasayanas* of Ayurvedic medicine, those herbal and mineral preparations used specifically for the purposes of physical regeneration rather than for the cure of disease.[5]

One of the more significant contributions of complementary medicine in the present time is its reminder that the work of the physician not only calls for the effective treatment of diseases, but also for the active support of health.

The freedom to choose

The health-based paradigm of complementary medicine has been strongly welcomed by many within Western communities. People are keen to learn what they can do to maintain their own and their families' wellbeing. The clinical style of the modalities of complementary medicine offers a highly personalised means whereby patients can become more informed in matters of health. The clinical encounter serves not only to provide relief for the patient's symptoms or condition, but also provides an opportunity to explore preventative and restorative strategies that the patient can work with in their own time.

The increasing presence and accessibility of practitioners prepared to work with patients in this way has been felt at all levels. An osteopath observes:

> Our local GP down the road here, who is very sound in her orthodox medicine, has sent a letter round to her patients saying now what times she is available and so on. She's doing a bit more advertising, and she also says in her letter that she is happy to work with alternative practitioners on people's problems. And so within the demographics of this area, patients are beginning to become sort of therapy shoppers who will have a number of different practitioners they go to for different things. And the GP, the medical GP is feeling the strain of that. She's not getting the people to come and consult her first.

This comment made in the mid-1990s reflects the reality on the ground for practitioners of biomedicine in a large Australian city. This scenario closely mirrors the situation in most English speaking countries throughout the world at the time. The expansion of the health care marketplace is not only a notable social and political phenomenon, but also carries significant economic implications. Even in crude terms, the increasing popularity of non-orthodox approaches to health care has resulted in greater competition between providers.

The increasing willingness of medical practitioners to cooperate with their non-medical colleagues may be driven as much by level-headed pragmatism as by a genuine desire for inter-professional conciliation and collaboration. Practitioners of biomedicine can no longer afford to alienate patients who have experienced for themselves the benefits of non-conventional approaches to health care.

Even during the 1980s, it was clear to some observers that the increasing popularity of non-orthodox healing modalities in the West carried strong implications for the direction in which the practice of community medicine was moving. Steven Fulder offered his own view of how things were shaping up in the United Kingdom at that time:

> The individuals concerned are ceasing to be mindless consumers of drugs and services, becoming more discriminating and aware in their choices. They are also bringing their new options back home to their family physicians, and contributing to an awareness among doctors of the existence and potential of natural therapies. It is the patients, rather than organised lobbies, who will bring about the coexistence and mutual respect between the various medical systems which is as obvious as it is inevitable.[6]

What was obvious and inevitable to Fulder at that time is rapidly coming to pass. One of the more significant consequences of this development is that many within biomedicine have extended their professional networks beyond the inner circle of specialist medical suites and now include the names of practitioners of complementary medicine on their patient referral lists. Practitioners across the board are beginning to talk to each other, and are becoming increasingly aware of the particular strengths and qualities of their respective approaches. In addition, many doctors are learning for themselves about ways of healing that may not have been part of their formal education through seminars, graduate programs and the pages of their professional journals.[7]

The core values of complementary medicine are reflected not so much in their unusual techniques or exotic pharmacopoeias, but in their expression of holistic principles. The disciplines themselves are characterised by a different relational style between patients and physicians to that of biomedicine. Their underlying philosophies tend to be health-based rather than disease-based. And the modalities of complementary medicine more comfortably accommodate the role of non-material influences in health and disease in their diagnostic and treatment methods.

Although there are strong currents of renewal coursing through medicine at present, the task of reclaiming the perennial values of physicianship is an historical one that cannot happen overnight. For behind many of the powerful institutions associated with biomedicine are particular interests that carry both their own momentum and their own inertia. Our osteopath continues:

> *The idea of psychosocial or psychosomatic medicine having something to say that would actually be heaps cheaper and heaps healthier won't really dawn on orthodox medicine ever because they make heaps more money . . . That probably always will be so. That high-tech, sexy, 'beyond 2000', physical, technological cure-type medicine—which actually never cures anything—will flourish. But the softer, more holistic approach will gather ground.*

Technology has reached into virtually every aspect of life in the developed world. The practice of biomedicine is no exception. The production of drugs, the manufacture and maintenance of diagnostic equipment, and the operation of acute and intensive care facilities, surgical theatres and nuclear medicine departments are all dependent on high technology. And although the perceived benefits of that technology may be great, this osteopath reminds us that they come at a cost, often a very high cost.

Huge amounts of money are vested in the discovery, manufacture and marketing of synthesised pharmaceutical drugs. And even greater amounts are generated by their sale. Our respondent reminds us of the obvious when he points out that such realities make it unlikely that things will change in a hurry.

The methods of complementary medicine do not require elaborate technologies and are generally far less costly than those of biomedicine. The correction of structural problems through manual methods will often eliminate the need for analgesic or anti-inflammatory medication. Herbal and homoeopathic medicines are easily produced from natural substances and are far less expensive than synthesised drugs. Disposable acupuncture needles can be carried anywhere and cost very little. Supplying the kitchen with whole foods costs little more, and often less, than their equivalent in processed and denatured foods, yet may provide health benefits for the whole family that are reflected in fewer episodes of sickness and a decreased need for medication.

Many sicknesses can be handled in ways other than the preferred methods of biomedicine and often at a fraction of the cost. The effective treatment of lifestyle-related or chronic degenerative diseases may require more than the setting and monitoring of drug schedules. The development of social support networks, and the cultivation of mental attitudes that enable a person better to deal with pain or limitation have a major role in the management of such conditions. So also does the facilitation of changes in patients' lifestyle and pattern of activities.

The osteopath quoted earlier seems quietly confident that despite the immense capabilities of technological medicine, 'the softer, more holistic approach will gather ground'. That ground has certainly been gained more recently. The very urgency of the times has called for a transcendence of the hostilities that, during the latter decades of the twentieth century, defined the boundaries of acceptable medicine. The old divisions now begin to give way to an increasingly integrated understanding.

The best and the worst of times

The scientific and technological developments of the past century have completely altered the way that humanity lives upon the earth. Machines now fly across continents and between planets. Our voices are invisibly carried through the ether by microwave radiation. Acts of war are perpetrated with deadly precision and devastating consequence by remote control. Five hundred million computers, all of which will eventually need to be disposed of, hum away in numerous households, businesses and institutions around the world. The cities of the earth are filled with the quiet roar of six hundred million cars as commuters daily brave peak hour.

During that same time, the remaining forests of northern Europe and North America have begun to wither under a rain of industrial pollutants. The skin of young children now reddens and blisters even under cloudy skies as the earth's protective ozone shield thins out. Southern icebergs the size of entire countries fracture and float northwards through shipping lanes. Majestic tropical coral reefs whiten and slowly die as the oceans begin to warm. Sixty-five million tons of precious topsoil is dispersed and lost every year through the methods of broadacre farming and contemporary agriculture. Elected politicians ignore calls to preserve old growth and tropical forests as ancient watchers of time are felled and turned to pulp and woodchip.

Our ways are strangely set in a peculiar yet understandable attachment to the hard-won benefits of industrial civilisation. It is as though we believe that we have either gone too far and can do little about the situation, or that if we just keep on with it, things will eventually sort themselves out. But there is a growing realisation that things are unlikely to sort themselves out of their own accord.

The intelligence and ingenuity that contributed to the creation of our present freedoms needs to turn not only towards minimising and repairing the damage that has already been done, but also towards developing a deeper understanding of how it is that such catastrophic harm has been allowed to go as far as it has.

Like the human body, the earth itself cannot be subjected to a constant and relentless assault without being severely damaged. As the health of the earth's finely balanced ecosystems is weakened through a progressive poisoning of air, water and the soil, so also is the health of the earth's inhabitants.[8]

The boiling frog principle

There is a story told that may give pause regarding the nature of the situation within which we presently find ourselves. If frogs are placed into a vat of water, they will swim happily about. If the water is gradually heated up, they will tend to swim a little faster. As the temperature steadily rises, they will swim more and more vigorously, but make no attempt to remove themselves from the increasingly dangerous environment in which they find themselves. One could say that they were adapting well to their changed circumstances. They adapt so well, in fact, that they will allow themselves to be eventually boiled to death. But if the same frogs are dropped into a vat of water that has already been heated to a high temperature, they will thrash and struggle fiercely in order to remove themselves from the deadly situation into which they have been placed.[9]

We have perhaps too vigorously defended the benefits of economic growth and technological development without giving sufficient attention to the more damaging consequences of such activities upon the biosphere and the earth's ecosystems, and upon human health. The very term 'diseases of civilisation' itself points to the known consequences of affluent and wasteful lifestyles.

The philosophy of holism rests on an understanding that all things are interconnected and that nothing occurs in isolation. For the first time in history, we know ourselves to be inhabitants of a finite world with finite resources, in a world that has been brought to its present state of equilibrium through hundreds of millions of years of slow adaptation to changing conditions. The past two centuries of human activity have brought about a degree of change in the natural balance of the world that could never have been fully anticipated. Many have become aware that the health of the earth's atmosphere, and of its terrestrial and marine ecosystems, is now in jeopardy. These changes herald difficult times ahead.

Ironically, it has been technology itself that has brought to our attention the true nature of our present predicament. The image of the earth from space represents one of the most powerful and transformative symbols in human consciousness. This image has made us all aware that we inhabit a single earth as one of myriad species that have arisen through the creative expression of the living forces of nature. Yet our industrial and commercial activities over the past two centuries have changed the balance of the earth's regulatory systems in ways we are barely beginning to come to terms with.

Cultural historian Thomas Berry has offered a profoundly disquieting assessment of the planetary consequences of industrial proliferation and its multiple influences upon the earth and its myriad ecosystems:

> The earth cannot sustain such an industrial system or its devastating tech-nologies. In the future, the industrial system will have its elements of apparent recovery, but these will be minor and momentary. The larger movement is towards dissolution. The impact of our present technologies is beyond what the earth can endure.[10]

One year after Berry offered this judgement regarding the present situation, the Union of Concerned Scientists issued a statement entitled 'World Scientists' Warning to Humanity'. It included the following comment:

> A great change in our stewardship of the earth and the life on it is required if vast human misery is to be avoided and our home on this planet is not to be irretrievably mutilated.[11]

These are not the hysterical projections of latter-day Luddites, but represent sober assessments of present realities. The Union of Concerned Scientists' Warning was endorsed by over 1700 of the world's leading scientists, in-cluding the majority of Nobel laureates in the sciences.

Thomas Berry has devoted most of his adult life to a study of human history and its various cultural manifestations. In recent decades, his energies have been directed towards understanding the nature of human connected-ness with the earth, and pursuing the deeper meaning of twentieth-century technological civilisation. Now in his nineties, Berry continues his work as an advocate for a more holistic and conscious cooperation with the forces that sustain all of life on the planet. Berry believes that our present predicament has been brought about through a growing separation from nature and natural forces that has occurred over the past three centuries. He attributes this desacralisation and loss of communion with the earth to the widespread influence of Descartes' dualistic philosophy upon the scientific community.[12]

The work ahead will require more than elaborate recycling systems and a reduction of the amount of energy that we consume, although these are essential elements of any program that seeks to limit further damage. The healing of the earth will be accomplished not so much by developing new technical solutions to the present problems, but by becoming more conscious of our integral relatedness to each other and to the earth and by acting accordingly. We are a part of nature and not apart from nature, and will inevitably suffer the consequences of any disturbance we may cause, whether individually or collectively, to natural systems.

The growth of interest in complementary medicine that occurred during the latter decades of the twentieth century needs to be understood in the broader context of such realities.

Recovering nature

Complementary medicine has not arisen in a vacuum. Even though its various modalities have been quietly practised alongside biomedicine throughout the early and middle decades of the twentieth century, there occurred a dramatic growth in the popularity in what was then referred to as 'alternative' or 'natural' medicine during the 1960s and 1970s. This appeared to be part of a wide-ranging cultural response to the escalating problems confronting contemporary civilisation. Those problems included increasing environmental degradation, rampant consumerism, a growing nuclear militarism and widespread social alienation.[13]

The growth of both the holistic health movement and the rise of alternative or complementary medicine have been linked to the development of what became known as the counter-culture during the 1960s. In the United States, nursing educator Kristine Alster observed:

> Although holistic thought has a long tradition in many disciplines, including medicine, it was the counter-culture that was the direct antecedent of the holistic health movement.[14]

This notion was more recently revisited by British sociologist Mike Saks. He suggested that the ideas and the consciousness that were identified with the counter-culture movement of the 1960s were significant influences in the growth in popularity of 'alternative' systems of medicine at the time:

> Although there had been an undercurrent of public scepticism about medical orthodoxy since its establishment in both Britain and the United States, what was different about the mid-1960s was the scale and intensity with which this was manifested. The emergence of a strong medical counter-culture was also importantly associated with the wider social changes that were taking place in the West . . .

> [T]he long-standing materialistic values that emphasised the delivery
> of technocratic solutions to problems generally came under fire at this
> time. The ideology of 'scientific progress' was also debunked, as growing
> numbers of the public sought to escape from established patterns of
> deference to authority and to explore alternative lifestyles.[15]

What is now commonly referred to as complementary medicine is more in
the nature of a social and cultural phenomenon than simply a group of
competing systems of therapy jousting for a place in the health care arena.
This development is characterised by a number of distinctive attributes: a
higher value tends to be placed on the natural world than the man-made
world; self-reliance is valued over dependence, interconnectedness over sep-
arateness, sustainability over consumerism, and cooperation over competition.
Support for the environment movement, the peace movement and an interest
in spirituality and the wisdom traditions of indigenous cultures are also
common elements within this development.

The high level of community support for the modalities of complementary medicine represents but one manifestation of the sense that our lives
have somehow lost touch with the deeper realities within which we participate, consciously or unconsciously. More holistic approaches to health care
offer a means of partially reclaiming those realities. A naturopath offers her
own reflection:

> I suppose it's something to do with the advance of science and technol-
> ogy and the whole worship of that in modern life. We're getting further
> and further away from a natural state and more and more into a techno-
> logical artificial world. Medicine's a big part of that. And what alternative
> medicine is trying to bring back or maintain is the natural, or some
> elements of the natural world.

It has already been noted that, in contrast to biomedicine, the modalities of
complementary medicine are relatively independent of high technology.
Within the Australian context, the term natural medicine was generally used
up until the 1990s to describe such approaches as naturopathy, homoeopathy, herbalism, many of the manual therapies and mind–body medicine.
This term points towards a major difference in perception of both the
methods and the philosophies of complementary medicine and biomedicine.
Rightly or wrongly, the modalities of complementary medicine are perceived
to be more closely linked with the natural world, while biomedicine and its
institutions are perceived to be part of the technological world.

The living forces that drive a seed to its full expression as a mature plant,
and the mysterious processes that transform a caterpillar into a butterfly are

manifestations of the same powers that sustain our own human nature. Our foods when wisely used become as medicines, and there are also within nature many plants that are capable of acting as agents for the healing of our sicknesses. The energy carried in a high-potency homoeopathic medicine and the intention carried in human caring and the healing touch can similarly act as forces for healing.

The naturopath quoted above sees the dependence of biomedicine upon technology as a source of alienation not only between doctors and patients, but also between medicine itself and the forces that sustain our life and our health. She points towards what Thomas Berry has called the technological 'entrancement' that can blind us to a perception of the natural world as a perennial repository of healing influences and capabilities.

This perspective in many ways goes against the temper of the times and the view that technology is a universally positive source of human progress and material abundance. The diagnostic technologies of biomedicine certainly represent an expression of extraordinary creativity and immense usefulness. But the shadow cast by industrial technologies over the past century appears to be darkening our collective futures as environmental degradation, deforestation, rising levels of greenhouse gasses, loss of the protective ozone layer and increasing levels of background radiation all continue to gather momentum.

The philosophies and practices underlying the modalities of complementary medicine remind us of the existence of perennial forms and perennial values within healing that transcend the particular circumstances of any given era. Nature remains capable of producing medicines without the manipulation by pharmaceutical engineers of atoms within and around complex molecules under conditions of high temperature and pressure. The skilled use of our hands will often help overcome joint restriction and inflammation far more decisively than measured doses of analgesics or anti-inflammatory drugs. And inner motivation or change may prove to be of far greater influence than outer intervention in the task of reclaiming and restoring health. A practitioner of traditional Chinese medicine reflects:

> I think that health, the secrets of health are locked up in nature. And I think this is probably why most of us are, why a majority of people are so ill, because of our so-called civilised living. I'm not sure that civilisation has done all that much good for man, to be quite honest.

This comment reiterates the view that the present age has somehow seen a profound loss in our relationship with the world of nature. The natural world has been treated as a commodity that exists largely for our own benefit. Until recently, there has been but little regard for the damage that has been wrought upon the earth and its ecosystems through industrial, commercial, military and agricultural activities. The natural cycles that exert a subtle influence upon living processes have also been largely overridden by our 'civilised' lifestyles. Our foods are transported across continents and between hemispheres regardless of the season. Our eating patterns are determined more by coffee and lunch breaks than by hunger. And our minor sicknesses are treated with drugs rather than by rest and recuperation.

The world view of this practitioner is conditioned by a Chinese medical philosophy that draws from Taoist understandings of our connectedness with the timeless cycles and rhythms of the natural world. Medical researcher and historian Rene Dubos reflects further:

> Biological rhythms were inscribed in man's genetic make-up during evolutionary development when human life was closely linked to the natural events determined by the movements of the earth around the sun and of the moon around the earth. Biological rhythms are important for the understanding of modern man because they persist even though he now lives in an artificial environment. He may intellectually forget diurnal, lunar and seasonal influences, but he cannot escape their physiological and mental effects.[16]

Even though technology has enabled us to live for extended periods of time cruising the ocean floor in submarines carrying multiple nuclear warheads, and to wheel beyond the earth's atmosphere in space shuttles that place new satellite systems into orbit, we yet remain part of nature.

Despite the awesome capabilities of technology, we continue to be influenced by the rhythms within nature that have been created through aeons of adaptation and evolutionary change. Technology has enabled us to transcend the limits of the natural world in ways that have never before been possible. In the process, we have also changed the character of the natural world to a mythic extent. Species extinction, loss of biodiversity, desertifi-cation and climate change are but part of the cost of this extraordinary dance with power.

There is a growing sense that our Promethean fire may engulf rather than kindle, may destroy rather than transform, and that we should return our attention to the earth from which we were formed and from which are derived our perennial sources of renewal.

The opening doors

The growth of complementary medicine has brought about a realisation that healing is a multidimensional phenomenon that can be approached from many directions. The range of modalities of complementary medicine attests to this reality. As the biomedical mind-set itself begins to move beyond reductionist philosophies and fixed patterns of treatment based largely upon pharmaceutical and surgical interventions, we witness an increasing receptivity to the forms that were not so long ago dismissed as spurious and ineffectual.

It is no longer unusual to find biomedical practitioners using or recommending acupuncture, spinal manipulation, vitamins and minerals, herbal medicines or psychosomatic approaches such as meditation and deep relaxation. The mind of biomedicine has begun to awaken to a deeper understanding of the complexity of our natures, and to the realisation that healing can occur in ways that are not necessarily taught in medical school. An acupuncturist reflects:

> People can't live by the biomedical methods alone. There need to be people who are skilled at working at the earth levels, working with things like herbs, and using the natural sort of products of the world that have been provided here to help us maintain this balance. And there need to be people that can work with their hands, who can work with people at that tactile level. There need to be people who are well trained to be able to work at energetic levels. There need to be people that can work at the heart to heart level. There need to be people that can work at the spiritual and philosophical levels. They all need to be there.

We have here a quintessential statement of the task that lies ahead. The significance of biomedicine is fully acknowledged. But the value of the many other forms of healing is also poetically affirmed. The earth itself produces our medicinal plants and nourishing foods and is honoured as a great source of healing influences that can be effectively brought to the task of healing. The importance of skilled touch, whether it takes the form of structural diagnosis and correction, of comfort and reassurance, or as a direct source of healing energy, is similarly honoured.

Beyond the nourishment, repair and restoration of our physical bodies, our energetic natures may also be harmonised and strengthened through the influence of those whose vision or sensitivity is tuned to the more subtle realms of consciousness. The importance of love, relationship, compassion and empathy in the work of true healing is reaffirmed.

This quote further reminds us that our souls and spirits may need as much nourishment and restoration and healing as our bodies during times of difficulty, of grief, or of collapse of meaning in our lives. The call to physicianship needs to embrace the full extent of human pain and suffering and attend to our total humanity, not just our physical embodiment.

Towards the future

As we draw towards a conclusion, it may be helpful to reflect back and bring together as far as possible the central notions that underlie this work.

It is clear that the will to heal is indelibly imprinted in our natures. This is reflected in the capacity of all living organisms for self-repair and restoration after injury and sickness. And this is more poignantly expressed in the human desire to help and care for others in their times of sickness and suffering.

Throughout history, this desire has given rise to many creative responses. The prayers and intercessions of the shaman, the compounding of medicines from the products of nature, the manipulation of body energies through touch and through the medium of acupuncture needles, and the activation of both the human will and the capacity of the body to renew itself through fasting or dietary restriction are all manifestations of the desire to alleviate the suffering borne of sickness, and to restore a state of health and wholeness.

The earlier chapters of this text have hopefully offered an appreciation of the relativity of healing practices and deepened our awareness of the human ingenuity that has constantly sought to overcome limitation and uncertainty. Reviewing the various forms that healing has taken at different times and in different places will also better enable us to view contemporary Western medicine as part of a broader historical project that continues to change and evolve.

There is a potency today that is unique in human history. Some view our present state of knowledge and technological mastery as an omega point of sorts, an epiphany towards which all of history has been moving, and the culmination of all previous human aspiration. But others, while acknowledging the immense creativity embodied in contemporary technological civilisation, view present developments as relative and contingent expressions that have been won through the negation of earlier accomplishments, and at the cost of a potentially ruinous disregard of both existential and environmental consequences.

Regardless of what position one may hold, it has become clear that we live in a nodal time, a time of great change, a time that has been described by physicist and cultural critic Fritjof Capra as a turning point upon which our collective future pivots.

It is in this light that the present changes occurring in the practice of medicine in the West should be seen. Although Jan Smuts coined the term 'holism' less than a century ago, holistic principles have informed the human understanding for thousands of years. The application of these principles was evident in the medicine of ancient Egypt and Greece, and continues to underlie many Eastern and traditional systems of medicine in the present day.

Throughout the time that rational scientific epistemologies have progressively altered the knowledge base, shaped the education style and determined the clinical standards of biomedicine, the modalities of complementary medicine have quietly carried the holistic understandings that had been largely overshadowed by the great successes of a new scientific medicine based upon reductionist principles. These holistic understandings were based upon a synthetic rather than an analytic approach to matter, life and mind. They were reflected in a therapeutic approach that placed a high value on the relationship between physician and patient, and that sought to enlist in whatever manner possible the inherent healing capacities of the patient.

The presence of complementary medicine is now well established within Western communities. It is supported by numerous patients, is increasingly attracting the attention of many students and educators within biomedicine and, as evidenced by the entry of many of its modalities into university environments, has won the active support of policy makers. There is no turning back. What is the true significance of this phenomenon? What are the likely consequences of this extraordinary social development in the lives of those who take on the role of healer and those who seek out their services? What does this mean for the future of medicine?

The holistic sensitivity accepts that human reality includes our physical bodies, our mental capacities and our spiritual aspirations. It also recognises that we are integrally connected with each other, with the natural and man-made world, and with the subtle energetic fields within which we live, move and have our being.

As holistic understandings begin to be more widely explored and accepted by those who would become healers, the practice of medicine will inevitably change in character. Many of those quoted throughout this text offer substantive insight into how the application of holistic principles can find expression in a therapeutic environment.

Although there will always be a place for the more powerful technological elements within biomedicine, particularly in such areas as diagnostic testing, surgery and emergency medicine, there is yet much work to be done in developing a deeper knowledge of how patients can be helped to help themselves in their own healing. The presently clearly marked boundaries between physician and patient may well begin to soften with the realisation that ultimately, we are to become our own healers.

A growing realisation of the reality of interconnectedness will necessarily broaden the base of medicine from its present predominantly personal and biological focus to one that further encompasses the role of mental influences, social pressures and environmental realities on our health. This in turn will bring to attention the fact that individual health is but one facet of the radiant jewel that constitutes living reality. Our own health cannot be separated from that of our families, our communities and of the planet itself.

The rise of complementary medicine, and the holism that it embodies, in recent times represents, among other things, a healing force within the healing profession itself. It offers perspectives that can provide balance for a system of medicine that has become highly dependent upon increasingly expensive technological interventions in the treatment of disease. It offers a timely and needed reminder that the work of the physician needs to embrace not only a mastery of disease and its treatment, but also an equally deep knowledge of the nature of health, and the many means whereby it may be actively supported and strengthened.

The modalities of complementary medicine have already seeded the newly emerging landscape of twenty-first century medicine. Their influence will continue to nourish the desire for a restoration of the human dimension to the historical mission of medicine. They will continue to provide well-seasoned methods and insights for the creation of health-based paradigms of healing. And they will further the integration of holistic principles into our understanding of what medicine is and should be.

~

The ideas that have been explored in the preceding chapters represent an expression of many of the perennial values that have driven the mission of medicine regardless of time and place. These values call attention to principles that transcend the technical capabilities of any given era. They relate, rather, to the subtler dimensions of healing alluded to in such notions as the integrity of body and mind, our connection with natural forces and spiritual reality, and the power latent in healing relationships.

These ideas have been explored through the voices of representatives of a number of modalities of complementary medicine. Each of those represented both teaches and practises their chosen modality. As educators, they are committed to developing an articulate and communicable knowledge base of their respective discipline. As practitioners, they participate in the concerns and experiences of their patients, and are witness to both the effectiveness and limitations of their own particular approach. Operating outside of the biomedical mainstream, they are also privy to the frustrations and disappointments of many who have sought and failed to find hoped-for relief of their symptoms and conditions through more conventional means.

Despite the great diversity in their training and educational experiences, there is consistent agreement regarding the central differences between their own approach and that which they identify as being more characteristic of biomedicine. It is hoped that the notions discussed throughout the preceding chapters do honour to the depth of thought and genuineness of intention of each respondent.

Those who have served as educators in the arena of complementary medicine, particularly during the latter decades of the twentieth century, have done so with a keen awareness of the historic nature of their activity. Their work was accomplished with very little institutional support, and was long overshadowed by the marginality of their position within health care. Yet their constancy and perseverance enabled the progressive creation of an informed and competent body of practitioners whose healing work within the community has sounded far more loudly than any polemic.

The dedication of generations of practitioners who have quietly worked outside of the biomedical mainstream, often under suspicion and disdain, has borne its own fruit in the present day. As the spirit of holism begins to infuse the practice of medicine in the Western world, we come ever closer to that healing that is needed at all levels. The wheel of medicine now turns towards a commitment to those principles that further the health of individuals, of society, and of the planet as a whole.

Glossary

Alchemy: The precursor to chemistry. Alchemy is based upon the notion that entities within the animal, vegetable and mineral kingdoms consist of body, soul and spirit. Its historical aims included the transmutation of metals and the preparation of medicines.

Arationality: Beyond, or outside of rationality. Arationality differs from irrationality in that it transcends rather than contradicts rational processes.

Arcana: A term often used by early chemists to describe the active principles hidden within matter.

Biomedicine: That form of medicine developed in the Western world over the past century which is based largely on the biological sciences. The term is used synonymously with 'Western medicine' and 'scientific medicine'.

Cartesian dualism: The philosophical position wherein matter and mind are viewed as separate entities. The concept was developed and popularised by the philosopher and mathematician René Descartes during the seventeenth century.

Chakra: The Sanskrit term for 'wheel'. In the yogic tradition, the term chakra is used to describe a number of energetic vortices or centres of spiritual power that are said to be located within the human body.

Ch'i: A Chinese term used to describe a bipolar energy said to circulate in the body through a series of meridians, or energetic conduits.

Colonic cleansing: A process whereby the contents of the large bowel are voided through the use of an enema or clyster. The method is popular among adherents of the hygienist tradition.

Consciousness: The faculty whereby one has awareness of both the inner world of thoughts, feelings and imagination, and the outer world of action, events and phenomena.

Depth interview: One of the methods of qualitative research that enables one to gain knowledge of the lived world of another. Depth interview techniques involve recording, transcription and analysis of focused discussions with a view to gaining a global impression of the concerns or understandings of individuals and of social groups.

Doctrine of specific aetiology: The theory that all diseases have a specific cause. This idea gained currency during the nineteenth century as a result of the development of bacteriology and the germ theory of disease. It was dramatically furthered by the development of endocrinology, and an understanding of the nature of diseases caused by hormone deficiency.

Empathy: The capacity to identify with the feelings and understandings of others. Through empathic engagement, one is able to participate in, and hence better understand, the lived experience of another.

Empiricism: An approach to knowledge based more upon observation and experiment than upon theoretical considerations. Empirical approaches ultimately rest on the experience of the senses rather than adherence to theory.

Epidemiology: The study of the incidence of disease and patterns of disease within human populations. Epidemiological studies are undertaken in order to understand both how diseases are transmitted through human groups, and in order to develop ways of controlling disease based on that understanding.

Epistemology: That branch of philosophy concerned with the nature of knowledge, the ways whereby knowledge of phenomena may be gained, and the basis for determining the validity of that knowledge.

Explication: The act of interpreting or detailing the various aspects or dimensions of a given phenomenon in order that its meaning may be better understood.

Gestalt: The German word for 'form' or 'shape'. The term is commonly used to describe a unified or integrated patterning or configuration that functions as a whole.

Hegemony: A term used to describe the dominance or undue influence of one particular group over other groups.

Hieratic: A term that describes priestly functions or sacred duties.

Holism: A philosophical position directed towards an understanding of wholes. The term, as used by its originator Jan Smuts in the early 1920s, incorporates the notion that the phenomenal world represents a unified expression of matter, mind and life. In relation to medicine, holism refers to an approach to treatment that is directed more towards the whole person than towards the disease or pathology with which they have been diagnosed.

Humoral theory: A traditional view of the influences that determine health and condition one's physical and mental tendencies. These influences were early described in the European tradition as blood, phlegm, black bile and yellow bile. They were said to correspond with sanguine, phlegmatic, melancholic and choleric temperaments. The humoral theory of health and disease formed a significant part of the medicine of Galen in the third century and continued to remain active in European medical thinking for over one and a half thousand years. Both traditional Chinese medicine and Ayurvedic medicine continue to make use of similar concepts.

Hygienism: An approach to health that builds strongly on the purist metaphor. Hygienist approaches emphasise the importance of pure and unprocessed foods in the maintenance of health and the use of periodic fasts and dietary restriction to eliminate toxins from the body.

Inherent healing: The capacity of the body for self-repair.

Magic bullet: A highly specific therapeutic agent capable of destroying the specific cause or causes of disease. The term has often been applied to those antibiotic agents that selectively target specific micro-organisms or groups of micro-organisms.

Materia medica: The Latin term for 'medicinal materials'. The term is commonly used to describe the remedial agents used in the various systems of herbal medicine and in homoeopathy.

Meridian: A conduit through which vital energies are said to circulate through the body according to traditional Chinese medicine. The purpose of acupuncture treatment is to harmonise the quality and flow of those energies through the needling of particular points.

Moxibustion: A form of treatment in traditional Chinese medicine based on the stimulation of acupuncture points with heat generated by the burning of small cones or sticks of compressed herbs. Most commonly, *Artemesia sinensis* is used, though other plants or their extracts may be added.

New physics: The post-Newtonian system of physics based on the interchangeability of matter and energy, the unitary nature of space and time, and the interconnectedness of everything within the universe.

Osteopathic lesion: A term used in osteopathic medicine to describe joint dysfunction.

Paradigm: The term coined by science historian Thomas Kuhn to describe ways of seeing the world that characterise particular discipline areas.

Participant observation: A method of research in the human sciences that is based on unintrusive participation in the life-world of a particular social group.

Placebo: A substance or procedure with no therapeutic value that is often used as a control in the testing of new drugs of therapeutic procedures.

Potencies (homoeopathic): The term used to describe the various attenuations or dilutions of the substances used in homoeopathic medicine.

Pragmatism: The principle of practicality. Pragmatic approaches tend to be more concerned with the feasibility and consequences of actions as they relate to particular circumstances than with adherence to principles or ideals.

Qualitative research: Methods of investigation of the natural world that are based on the identification and interpretation of qualities associated with given phenomena. Qualitative research methods are most commonly used in the social sciences.

Quantitative research: Methods of investigation based upon measurement, quantification and statistical analysis.

Reductionism: A philosophical position that holds that complex systems can best be understood by isolating and identifying their constituent elements or components.

Shamanism: A traditional cultural system based on the notion that the world is infused with spiritual energy with which certain individuals can directly engage. Central to the practice of shamanism is the shaman, who acts as mediator between the spirit world and the human world. The shaman serves not only as carrier of the myths and stories of his or her people, but often serves as healer.

Spirit: A non-material energetic principle that is said to animate living matter. Spirit is also understood to be part of a reality that is independent of matter.

Structural restriction: An osteopathic term used to describe a state of limited mobility in one or several of the bony joints of the human body.

Taoism: A religious philosophy originating in China that holds the universe to be an interconnected reality. Taoism places a high value on attaining a state of harmony with both the natural world and with the Divine order, or Tao.

Technocracy: A term used to describe those who seek to exert social and political control through technology and technical expertise.

Therapeutic touch: A term coined by nursing educator Dolores Krieger for an approach to healing based on the intentional transference of therapeutic energy from one person to another.

Trophorestoration: A term used in the Western herbal medicine tradition that describes the physiological restoration of damaged organs or organ systems through the use of plant medicines.

Vis medicatrix naturae: Latin term for the healing power of nature.

Vital force: The energetic principle that is said to sustain life.

Vitalism: A philosophical position that holds that life is sustained by an active non-material force different to those forces mediated by the processes associated with biochemistry and physiology.

References

Achterberg, J 1987, 'The Shaman: Master healer in the imaginary realm', in Shirley Nicholson (ed), *Shamanism: An expanded view of reality*, Theosophical Publishing House, Wheaton, Illinois.

Alster, K 1989, *The Holistic Health Movement*, University of Alabama Press, Tuscaloosa.

Bakx, K 1991, 'The "eclipse" of folk medicine in Western society', *Sociology of Health and Sickness*, vol. 13 (1), pp. 20–38.

Balint, M 1964, *The Doctor, His Patient and the Illness*, 2nd edn, Pitman Medical, London.

Barrett, B, Marchand, L et al 2004, 'What Complementary and Alternative Medicine Practitioners Say About Health and Health Care', *Annals of Family Medicine*, vol. 2, pp. 253–9.

Baum, M 1989, 'Rationalism versus Irrationalism in the Care of the Sick: Science versus the absurd', *Medical Journal of Australia*, vol. 151, p. 607.

Beecher, H 1966, 'Ethics and Clinical Research', *The New England Journal of Medicine*, vol. 274, 24, 1354–60.

Bell, I, Caspi, O et al 2002, 'Integrative Medicine and Systemic Outcomes Research: Issues in the emergence of a new model for primary health care', *Archives of Internal Medicine*, vol. 162(2), pp. 133–40.

Bensoussan, A 1999, 'Complementary medicine: where lies its appeal?', *Medical Journal of Australia*, vol. 170, 247–8.

Berliner, H 1984, 'Scientific Medicine since Flexner', in J.W. Salmon (ed), *Alternative Medicines: Popular and policy perspectives*, Tavistock, New York.

Berliner, H and Salmon, J 1980, 'The Holistic Alternative to Scientific Medicine: History and analysis', *International Journal of Health Services*, vol. 10, 1, 133–47.

Berman, B 2001, 'Complementary medicine and medical education: teaching complementary medicine offers a way of making teaching more holistic', *BMJ*, vol. 322: 121–2.

Berry, T 1991, *The Ecozoic Era* (Presented at 11th Annual E.F. Schumacher Lecture, October 1991, Great Barrington, Massachusetts). Viewed at <http://www.schumachersociety.org/lec-tber.html>

——1995, *The University: Its response to the ecological crisis*, Paper delivered before the University Committee on Environment, Harvard University, 11 April 1996. Viewed at <http://ecoethics.net/ops/univers.htm>

Bertell, R 1985, *No Immediate Danger: Prognosis for a radioactive earth*, The Women's Press, London.

Blumenthal, M, Busse, WR, Goldberg, A et al (eds) 1998, *The Complete Commission E Monographs: Therapeutic guide to herbal medicines*, American Botanical Council, Austin.

Boyers, R and Orrill, R 1972, *Laing and Anti-Psychiatry*, Penguin, Harmondsworth, United Kingdom.

British Herbal Pharmacopeia Parts 1–3 (1976–1981), British Herbal Medicine Association, Cowling, United Kingdom.

Brooks, P 2004, 'Undergraduate Teaching of Complementary Medicine', *MJA*, vol. 181 (5), p. 275.

Brown, ER 1979, *Rockefeller Medicine Men: Medicine and capitalism in America*, University of California Press, Berkeley.

Calabrese, C 2002, 'Clinical Research in Naturopathic Medicine', in Jonas, W, Lewith, G and Walach, H, *Clinical Research in Complementary Therapies. Principles, Problems and Solutions*, Churchill Livingstone London.

Capra, F 1982, *The Turning Point. Science, society and the rising culture*, Fontana edition, London.

Carlson, R 1975, *The End of Medicine*, John Wiley and Sons, New York.

Cassell, E 1976, *The Healer's Art*, MIT Press, Cambridge, Massachusetts.

Center for Defence Information 2003, *CDI Factsheet: Ricin*, Washington DC. Cited at <http://www.cdi.org/terrorism/ricin-pr.cfm>

Chojnowski, P, 'Descartes' Dream. From method to madness', *The Angelus*, XXV, no. 4, April 2002. Viewed at http://www.sspx.ca/Angelus/2002_May/Descartes.htm>

Cornaro, L 1903, *The Art of Living Long*, William F. Butler, Milwaukee.

Coulter, I and Willis, E 2004, 'The rise and rise of complementary and alternative medicine: a sociological perspective', *MJA*, vol. 180 (11): 587–9.

Council of Islamic Education, 'Contributions of Muslims to the Field of Medicine', pp. 177–86. Viewed at <www.cie.org/pdffiles/smpiren 3.pdf>

Dakin, HS 1975, *High Voltage Photography*, 2nd edn, H.S. Dakin, San Francisco.

Dash, VB 1978, *Fundamentals of Ayurvedic Medicine,* Bansal and Co., Dehli.

Dawson, WR 1929, *Magician and Leech: A study in the beginnings of medicine with special reference to ancient Egypt,* Methuen and Co., London.

Debus, A 1978, *Man and Nature in the Renaissance,* Cambridge University Press, Cambridge.

Di Stefano, V 1990, 'Towards Regeneration', *Australian Journal of Medical Herbalism,* vol. 2, 3, pp. 55–8

——1994, 'Paracelsus: Light of Europe' (Parts 1–3), *Australian Journal of Medicinal Herbalism,* vol. 6, 1, pp. 5–8.

——1996, 'Of Spirochetes and Rainforests: The search for new drugs', *Journal of the Australian Traditional Medicine Society,* vol. 2, 4, pp. 89–93

——1998, 'The Meaning of Natural Medicine: An interpretive study', M.H.Sc. thesis (unpublished), Department of Health Sciences, Victoria University, Melbourne.

Dobbs, B 1975, *The Foundations of Newton's Alchemy: or, 'The Hunting of the Greene Lyon',* Cambridge University Press, Cambridge.

Dormann, T 2004, 'Colonics. Forbidden Medicine', *Townsend Letter for doctors and patients.* Viewed at <http://www.townsendletter.com/July2004/colonics07 04.htm>

Dossey, L 1982, *Space, Time and Medicine,* Shambhala, Boulder.

——1993, *Healing Words: The power of prayer and the practice of medicine,* Harper Collins, San Francisco.

Dubois, J 1952, *The Devil's Chemists,* Beacon Press, Boston.

Dubos, R 1959, *Mirage of Health: Utopias, progress and biological change,* Anchor Books, New York.

——1979, 'Hippocrates in Modern Dress', in Sobel, D (ed), *Ways of Health: Holistic approaches to ancient and contemporary medicine,* Harcourt, Brace, Jovanovich, New York pp. 205–20.

Ehrenreich, J (ed) 1978, *The Cultural Crisis of Modern Medicine,* Monthly Review Press, New York.

Encyclopaedia Britannica 1927, *Holism and Science.*

Fairbanks, A (ed. and trans.) 1898, *Empedocles. Fragments and Commentary,* Book 1, verse 33, K. Paul, Trench, Trubner, London. Viewed at <http:// history.hanover.edu/texts/presoc/emp.htm>

Feuerstein, G 1987, *Structures of Consciousness: The genius of Jean Gebser. An introduction and critique,* Integral Publishing, Lower Lake, California.

Foss, L 1989, 'A Challenge to Biomedicine: A Foundations Perspective', *Journal of Medicine and Philosophy,* vol. 14, pp. 165–91.

Friedson, E 1988, *Profession of Medicine: A study of the sociology of applied knowledge,* Chicago Press, Chicago.

Fulder, S 1988, *The Handbook of Complementary Medicine,* Oxford University Press, Oxford.

Garrison, FH 1929, *An Introduction to the History of Medicine*, W.B. Saunders Co., Philadelphia.

Gawler, I 1984, *You Can Conquer Cancer*, Hill of Content Publishing, Melbourne.

Gebser, J 1949, *The Ever-Present Origin* (trans. Noel Barstad), Ohio University Press, Athens, Ohio.

German, G 1987, 'The Traditional and the Modern in the Practice of Medicine', in Joske, R and Segal, W (eds), *Ways of Healing*, Penguin, Australia.

Gerson, M 1958, *A Cancer Therapy: Results of fifty cases*, Totality Books, Del Mar, California.

Ghalioungui, P 1963, *Magic and Medical Science in Ancient Egypt*, Hodder and Stoughton, London.

Graham, H 1990, *Time, Energy and the Psychology of Healing*, Jessica Kingsley Publishers Ltd, London.

Great Books Online, *Trotula of Salerno*. Viewed at <http://www.malaspina.com /site/person_1140.asp>

Guba, E 1990, *The Paradigm Dialogue*, Sage Publications, Newbury Park, California.

Harkness, J, Lederer, S and Wikler, D 2001, 'Laying ethical foundations for clinical research', *Bulletin of the World Health Organization*, 79 (4), 365–72.

Hartmann, F 1973, *Paracelsus: Life and prophecies*, Rudolph Steiner Publications, New York.

The Harvard Working Group on New and Resurgent Diseases 1995, 'New and Resurgent Diseases: The failure of attempted eradication', *The Ecologist*, vol. 25, no. 1, January/February, pp. 21–6.Hare, R 1970, *The Birth of Penicillin and the Disarming of Microbes*, George Allen and Unwin, London.

Hasted, J 1981, *The Metal Benders*, Routledge and Kegan Paul, London.

Henry, S (ed) 1941, *Four Treatises of Theophrastus von Hohenheim Called Paracelsus*, Johns Hopkins Press, Baltimore.

Hopkins, N 2003, 'Four remanded on ricin terror charges as six more arrested', *The Guardian*, 14 January. Viewed at <http://www.guardian.co. uk/Print/0,3858,4582797,00.html>

Illich, I 1976, *Limits to Medicine: Medical nemesis. The expropriation of health*, Marion Boyars, London.

Jacobi, J 1951, *Paracelsus: Selected writings*, Routledge and Kegan Paul, London.

Jensen, B 1981, *Tissue Cleansing Through Bowel Management*, Jensen, Escondido.

Johnson, K 1975, *The Living Aura: Radiation field photography and the Kirlian effect*, Hawthorn Books, New York.

Joske, R and Segal, W (eds) 1987, *Ways of Healing*, Penguin, Australia.

Journal of the American Medical Association, 'Alternative Medicine', vol. 280 (18), pp. 1549–640.

Jung, C 1958, *The Undiscovered Self*, Routledge and Kegan Paul, London.

———1963, *Memories, Dreams and Reflections*, Collins and Routledge and Kegan Paul, London.

Kakar, S 1982, *Shamans, Mystics and Doctors: A psychological inquiry into India and its healing traditions*, University of Chicago Press, Chicago.

Kaptchuk, T 2002, 'The Placebo Effect in Alternative Medicine: Can the performance of a healing ritual have clinical significance?', *Annals of Internal Medicine*, vol. 136, pp. 817–25.

Karagulla, S 1967, *Breakthrough to Creativity*, De Vorss and Co., California.

Kleinman, A 1984, 'Indigenous Systems of Healing: Questions for professional, popular, and folk care', in Salmon, JW (ed), *Alternative Medicines: Popular and policy perspectives*, Tavistock, New York.

Kornberg, A 1987, 'The Two Cultures: Chemistry and Biology', *Biochemistry*, vol. 26, pp. 6888–891. Viewed at <http://www.uft.uni-bremen.de/chemie/isensee/kornberg_biochemistry.html>

Krieger, D 1979, *The Therapeutic Touch: How to use your hands to help and heal*, Prentice Hall, Englewood Cliffs, New Jersey.

Kuhn, T 1962, *The Structure of Scientific Revolutions*, University of Chicago Press, Chicago.

Laing, RD 1960, *The Divided Self*, Tavistock, New York.

———1961, *Self and Others*, Tavistock, New York.

Laing, RD and Esterton, A 1964, *Sanity, Madness and the Family*, Tavistock, New York.

Lane, E 1975, *Electrophotography*, And/Or Press, San Francisco.

Lewith, G, Jonas, W and Walach, H 2002, *Clinical Research in Complementary Therapies: Principles, problems and solutions*, Churchill Livingstone, London.

Lloyd, GE (ed) 1978, *Hippocratic Writings*, Penguin, London.

Lyons, AS and Petrucelli, RJ 1987, *Medicine: An illustrated history*, Abradale Press, New York.

Maizes, V and Caspi, O 1999, 'The principles and challenges of integrative medicine', *Western Journal of Medicine*, vol. 171, pp. 148–9.

Maizes, V, Schneider, C, Bell, I and Weil, A 2002, 'Integrative Medical Education: Development and implementation of a comprehensive curriculum at the University of Arizona', *Academic Medicine*, vol. 77, 9, pp. 851–60.

Marks, S 2000, *Jan Smuts, Race and the South African War*, SADOCC, Vienna. Viewed at <http://www.sadocc.at/publ/marks.pdf>

Matheson, C 1996, 'Historicist Theories of Rationality', *Stanford Encyclopaedia of Philosophy*. Viewed at <http://plato.stanford.edu/entries/rationality-historicist/>

May, R 1995, *The Art of Counselling*, Gardner Press, New York.

McGuire, M 1988, *Ritual Healing in Suburban America*, Rutgers University Press, New Brunswick.

McKenna, T and McKenna, D. 1975, *The Invisible Landscape*, Harper, San Francisco.

McKeown, T 1976, *The Role of Medicine: Dream, mirage, or nemesis?*, Nuffield Provincial Hospitals Trust, London.

McMichael, T 2002, 'The Biosphere, Health, and Sustainability' (editorial), *Science*, vol. 297, 16 August, p. 1093.

McWhinney, I 2001, 'Being a General Practitioner: What it means', *Primary Care*, vol. 1, 309–16.

Merton, T 1965, *Conjectures of a Guilty Bystander*, Sheldon Press, London.

Moss, D 1989, 'Psychotherapy and Human Experience', in Halling, S and Valle, R, *Existential-Phenomenological Perspectives in Psychology: Exploring the breadth of human experience*, Plenum, New York.

Mowrey, D 1986, *The Scientific Validation of Herbal Medicine*, Keats Publishing, Connecticut.

——1988, *Next Generation Herbal Medicine*, Keats Publishing, Connecticut.

Neville, B 1989, *Educating Psyche*, Collins Dove, Melbourne.

——1993, 'Five Kinds of Empathy', Paper presented to the third International Conference on Client-centred and Experiential Psychotherapy, Gmunden, Austria.

Newman, L 1999, 'Descartes' Epistemology, Section 7: Proving the existence of the external, material world', *Stanford Encyclopaedia of Philosophy*. Viewed at <http://www.plato.stanford.edu/entries/descartes-epistemology/>

Nicholson, S (ed) 1987, *Shamanism: An expanded view of reality*, Theosophical Publishing House, Wheaton, Illinois.

Pachter, H 1961, *Paracelsus: Magic into science*, Collier, New York.

Pagel, W 1958, *Paracelsus: An introduction to philosophical medicine in the era of the Renaissance*, S. Karger, Basel.

Pappworth, M 1967, *Human Guinea Pigs: Experimentation on man*, Routledge and Kegan Paul, London.

Pellegrino, E 1979, 'The Sociocultural Impact of Twentieth Century Therapeutics', in Rosenberg, E and Vogel, MD 1979, *The Therapeutic Revolution*, University of Pennsylvania Press, Philadelphia.

——1989, 'Towards an Expanded Medical Ethics: The Hippocratic ethic revisited', in Veach, R (ed), *Cross Cultural Perspectives in Medical Ethics: Readings*, Jones and Bartlett, Boston, p. 32.

Pelletier, K 1994, *Sound Mind, Sound Body: A new model for lifelong health*, Simon and Schuster, New York.

Peters, D (ed) 2001, *Understanding the Placebo Effect in Complementary Medicine*, Churchill Livingstone, London.

Pirotta, M, Cohen, M, Kitsirilos, V and Farish, S 2000, 'Complementary therapies: Have they become accepted in general practice?', *Medical Journal of Australia*, vol. 172, pp. 105–9.

Porkert, M 1979, 'Chinese Medicine: A traditional healing science', in

Sobel, D, *Ways of Health: Holistic approaches to ancient and contemporary medicine*, Harcourt, Brace, Jovanovich, New York.

Rees, L and Weil, A 2001, 'Integrated medicine', *British Medicial Journal*, vol. 322, pp. 119–20.

Reilly, D 2001, 'Some Reflections on Creating Therapeutic Consultations', in Peters, D (ed) 2001, *Understanding the Placebo Effect in Complementary Medicine*, Churchill Livingstone, London.

Remen, RN 1996, *Kitchen Table Wisdom: Stories that heal*, Pan Macmillan, Australia.

Renaud, M 1978, 'On the Structural Constraints to State Intervention in Health', in Ehrenreich, J (ed) 1978, *The Cultural Crisis of Modern Medicine*, Monthly Review Press, New York.

Riddle, M 1985, *Dioscorides on Pharmacy and Medicine*, University of Texas Press Austin.

Riva, A, *The History of Medicine*. Viewed at <http://pacs.unica.it/biblio/tocs.htm>

Robson, T (ed) 2003, *An Introduction to Complementary Medicine*, Allen & Unwin, Sydney.

Saks, M 2003, *Orthodox and Alternative Medicine: Politics, professionalization and health care*, Continuum Publishing Ltd, London.

Salmon, JW (ed) 1984, *Alternative Medicines: Popular and policy perspectives*, Tavistock, New York.

Schumacher, EF 1974, *Small is Beautiful: A study of economics as if people mattered*, Abacus, London.

Segal, W 1987, 'Naturopathy, Homeopathy and Herbalism', in Joske, R and Segal, W, *Ways of Healing*, Penguin, Melbourne, pp. 83–115.

Senfelder, L 1911, *A History of Medicine in the West*. Viewed at <http://www.newadvent.org/cathen/10122a.htm>

Sheldrake, R 1988, *The Presence of the Past: Morphic resonance and the habits of nature*, Collins, London.

Siegel, R 1968, *Galen's System of Physiology and Medicine*, S. Karger, Basel.

Sigerist, H (ed) 1941, *Four Treatises of Theophrastus von Hohenheim Called Paracelsus*, Johns Hopkins Press, Baltimore.

Silverman, B 2002, 'Monastic Medicine: A unique dualism between natural science and spiritual healing', *Harvard University Research Journal*, 1, 10–17. Viewed at <www.jhu.edu/hurj/issue1/Silverman_monasticMed/Silverman_monastic Med.pdf>

Singer, C and Underwood, EA 1962, *A Short History of Medicine*, Oxford University Press, Oxford.

Sivananda, S 1952, *Practice of Nature Cure*, Vigyan Press, Rishikesh.

Smith, R 2004, 'Foregone Conclusions: The public is being regularly deceived by the drug trials funded by pharmaceutical companies, loaded to generate the results they need', *The Guardian*, 14 January. Viewed at <http://www.guardian.co.uk/medicine/story/0,11381,1122721,00.html>

Smuts, J 1925, *Holism and Evolution*, Reprinted 1999, Sierra Sunrise Books, California (ed Sanford Holst).

Sobel, D (ed) 1979, *Ways of Health: Holistic approaches to ancient and contemporary medicine*, Harcourt, Brace, Jovanovich, New York.

Stacey, M 1988, *The Sociology of Health and Sickness*, Unwin, Hyman Ltd, London.

Starr, P 1949, *The Social Transformation of American Medicine*, Basic Books, New York.

Stein, H 1985, *The Psychodynamics of Medical Practice: Unconscious factors in patient care*, University of California Press, Berkeley.

Still, AT 1897, *Autobiography*, Kirksville. Repr. Maidstone Osteopathic Clinic, Maidstone.

Strauss, A and Corbin, J 1988, *Shaping a New Health Care System*, Jossey-Bass Inc., San Francisco.

Strehlow, W and Hertzka, G 1988, *Hildegard of Bingen's Medicine* (trans. Karin Strehlow), Bear and Co., Santa Fe.

Szasz, T 1961, *The Myth of Mental Illness* (revised edn, 1974), Harper and Row, New York.

Szasz, T and Hollander, M 1956, 'A Contribution to the Philosophy of Medicine: the Basic Models of the Doctor–Patient Relationship', *AMA Archives of Internal Medicine*, vol. 97, pp. 585–92.

Szekely, EB 1981, *The Essene Gospel of Peace: Book 1*, I.B.S. International, San Diego.

Taylor, R 1979, *Medicine Out of Control: The anatomy of a malignant technology*, Sun Books, Melbourne.

Thakkur, CJ 1974, *Ayurveda: The Indian art and science of medicine*, ASI Publishers, New York.

Toynbee, A 1976, *Mankind and Mother Earth*, Oxford University Press, Oxford.

Union of Concerned Scientists 1992, *World Scientists' Warning to Humanity*. Viewed at <http://www.ucsusa.org/ucs/about/page.cfm?pageID=1009>

Valle, R and Halling, S 1989, *Existential-Phenomenological Perspectives in Psychology: Exploring the breadth of human experience*, Plenum, New York.

Vincent, C and Furnham, A 1996, 'Why do patients turn to complementary medicine? An empirical study', *British Journal of Clinical Psychology*, vol. 35, pp. 37–48.

Vogel, MD and Rosenberg, CE 1979, *The Therapeutic Revolution*, University of Pennsylvania Press, Philadelphia.

Waite, AE 1894, *The Hermetic and Alchemical Writings of Paracelsus (Volumes I and II)*, Reprinted. 1976, Shambhala, Berkeley.

Wallach, H, Jonas, W and Lewith, G 2002, 'The Role of Outcomes Research in Evaluating Complementary Medicine', *Alternative Therapies*, vol. 8, 3, pp. 88–95.

Ward, B and Dubos, R 1972, *Only One Earth: The care and maintenance of a small planet*, W.W. Norton and Co., New York.

Wetzel, M, Eisenberg, D and Kaptchuk, T 1988, 'Courses Involving Complementary and Alternative Medicine at US Medical Schools', *Journal of the American Medical Association*, vol. 280, pp. 784-7.

Wetzel, M, Kaptchuk, T, Haramati, A and Eisenberg, D 2003, 'Complementary and Alternative Medical Therapies: Implications for medical education', *Annals of Internal Medicine*, vol. 138, 3, pp. 191–6.

Wilcox, B, Aguirre, A et al 2004, 'EcoHealth: A transdisciplinary imperative for a sustainable future' (Editorial), *EcoHealth*, vol. 1, pp. 3–5.

Withington, ET 1894, *Medical History from the Early Times*, Reprinted 1964 The Holland Press, London.

Zollman, C and Vickers, A 1999, 'ABC of Complementary Medicine: What is complementary medicine?', *British Medical Journal*, vol. 319, pp. 693–6.

Notes

Introduction

1. G Allen German, 'The Traditional and the Modern in the Practice of Medicine', in R Joske and W Segal (eds), *Ways of Healing*, pp. 13–28.
2. Arthur Kleinman, 'Indigenous Systems of Healing: Questions for professional, popular, and folk care', in JW Salmon (ed), *Alternative Medicines: Popular and policy perspectives*, p. 156.
3. Paul Starr, *The Social Transformation of American Medicine*, pp. 110–24; Margaret Stacey, *The Sociology of Health and Sickness*, pp. 76–99.
4. Jan Christian Smuts, *Holism and Evolution*.
5. 'Holism and Science', *Encyclopaedia Britannica*.
6. Jan Smuts, op. cit., pp. 150–7, 311–39.
7. Shula Marks, *Jan Smuts, Race and the South African War*, SADOCC, Vienna. Viewed at <http://www.sadocc.at/publ/marks.pdf>
8. Joe Pizzorno, 'Foreword' (p. x) in Terry Robson (ed), *An Introduction to Complementary Medicine*.
9. Victoria Maizes and Opher Caspi, 'The principles and challenges of integrative medicine', *West. J. Med.*, 1999, vol. 171, pp. 148–9; Lesley Rees and Andrew Weil, 'Integrated medicine', *BMJ*, 2001, vol. 322, pp. 119–20.
10. Miriam Wetzel, David Eisenberg, Ted Kaptchuk, 'Courses Involving Complementary and Alternative Medicine at US Medical Schools', *JAMA*, 1998, vol. 280, pp. 784–7; Marie Pirotta, Marc Cohen, Vicki Kotsirilos and Stephen Farish, 'Complementary therapies: Have they

become accepted in general practice?', *MJA*, 2000, vol. 172, pp. 105–9; Brian Berman, 'Complementary medicine and medical education: teaching complementary medicine offers a way of making teaching more holistic', *BMJ*, 2001, vol. 322, pp. 121–2.

11. Keith Bakx, 'The "eclipse" of folk medicine in Western society', *Sociology of Health and Sickness*, 1991, vol. 13 (1), pp. 20–38; Charles Vincent and Adrian Furnham, 'Why do patients turn to complementary medicine? An empirical study', *Br. J. Clin. Psychol.*, 1996, vol. 35, pp. 37–48; Bruce Barrett, Lucille Marchand et al, 'What Complementary and Alternative Medicine Practitioners say About Health and Health Care', *Annals of Family Medicine*, 2004, vol. 2, pp. 253–9.

12. Alan Bensoussan, 'Complementary medicine: where lies its appeal?', *MJA*, 1999, vol. 170, pp. 247–8; Ian Coulter and Evan Willis, 'The rise and rise of complementary and alternative medicine: a sociological perspective', *MJA*, 2004, vol. 180 (11), pp. 587–9.

13. Vincent Di Stefano 1998, 'The Meaning of Natural Medicine: An interpretive study', M.H.Sc. thesis (unpublished).

14. Bernie Neville 1993, *Five Kinds of Empathy*, Paper presented to the third International Conference on Client-centred and Experiential Psychotherapy', Gmunden, Austria, September 1994. See also his *Educating Psyche*.

Chapter I

1. David Sobel, 'Ancient Systems of Medicine', in David Sobel, *Ways of Health: Holistic approaches to ancient and contemporary medicine*, p. 107.

2. Eric Cassell, *The Healer's Art*, p. 222.

3. Paul Ghalioungui 1963, *Magic and Medical Science in Ancient Egypt*, pp. 41–3.

4. Ibid., pp. 70–3.

5. Quoted in Fielding H Garrison, *An Introduction to the History of Medicine*, p. 58.

6. Edmund Bordeaux Szekely, *The Essene Gospel of Peace: Book 1*, I.B.S. International; Sivananda, S, *Practice of Nature Cure*, Vigyan Press, Rishikesh; Thakkur, CJ, *Ayurveda: The Indian art and science of medicine*.

7. Bernard Jensen, *Tissue Cleansing Through Bowel Management*; Max Gerson, *A Cancer Therapy. Results of Fifty Cases*; see also Thomas Dorman, 'Colonics. Forbidden Medicine', *Townsend Letter for Doctors and Patients*. Viewed at <http://www.townsendletter.com/July2004/colonics0704.htm>

8. Warren R Dawson, *Magician and Leech: A study in the beginnings of medicine with special reference to ancient Egypt*, pp. 102–8.

9. Ibid., p. 116.

10. Nick Hopkins, 'Four remanded on ricin terror charges as six more arrested', *The Guardian*, 14 January 2003. Viewed at <http://www.guardian.co.uk/Print/0,3858,4582797,00.html>
11. Center for Defense Information 2003, *CDI Factsheet: Ricin*, Washington DC. Viewed at <http://www.cdi.org/terrorism/ricin-pr.cfm>
12. Quoted in Edward T Withington, *Medical History from the Early Times*, p. 46.
13. Diodorus Siculus, quoted in Paul Ghalioungui, op. cit., p. 107–8.
14. Arthur Fairbanks, *Empedocles. Fragments and Commentary*.
15. Quoted in Edward T Withington, op. cit., p. 54.
16. GE Lloyd, *Hippocratic Writings*. See 'Tradition in Medicine', pp. 70–86; 'Aphorisms', section IV, pp. 216–17.

Chapter 2

1. Walter Pagel, *Paracelsus: An Introduction to Philosophical Medicine in the Era of the Renaissance*, p. 144.
2. Fielding Garrison, *An Introduction to the History of Medicine*, p. 7.
3. John M. Riddle, *Dioscorides on Pharmacy and Medicine*, pp. 3–5.
4. Ibid., p. xvii.
5. Rudolph Siegel, *Galen's System of Physiology and Medicine*, p. 12.
6. Alessandro Riva, *The History of Medicine*.
7. AS Lyons, and RJ Petrucelli, *Medicine: An illustrated history*.
8. Leopold Senfelder, *A History of Medicine in the West*, p. 6.
9. Great Books Online, *Trotula of Salerno*.
10. Allen Debus, *Man and Nature in the Renaissance*, pp. 63–4; *see also* Leopold Senfelder, op. cit., p. 21.
11. Allen Debus, op. cit., p. 10.
12. Henry Pachter, *Paracelsus: Magic into science*, p. 57.
13. Ibid., p. 123.
14. Jolande Jacobi, *Paracelsus: Selected writings*, p. liii.
15. Ibid., p. lv.
16. Henry Pachter, op. cit., p. 186.
17. See Benjamin Silverman, 'Monastic Medicine: A unique dualism between natural science and spiritual healing'. *See also* Wighard Strehlow and Gottfried Hertzka, *Hildegard of Bingen's Medicine*.

Chapter 3

1. Elliott Friedson, *Profession of Medicine: A study of the sociology of applied knowledge*, p. 5.

2. Mike Saks, *Orthodox and Alternative Medicine: Politics, professionalization and health care*, p. 6.
3. Paul Starr, *The Social Transformation of American Medicine*, p. 42.
4. Howard Berliner and J Warren Salmon, 'The Holistic Alternative to Scientific Medicine: History and analysis', *International Journal of Health Services*, 1980, vol. 10, 1, 133–47, pp. 136–9. *See also* Leopold Senfelder, *A History of Medicine in the West*, pp. 32–9.
5. Margaret Stacey, *The Sociology of Health and Healing*, pp. 54–7.
6. Paul Starr, op. cit., p. 120.
7. ER Brown, *Rockefeller Medicine Men: Medicine and capitalism in America*, p. 192.
8. Paul Starr, op. cit., p. 7.
9. ER Brown, op. cit., pp. 84–91.
10. Ibid., p. 153.
11. Paul Starr, op. cit., p. 123.
12. ER Brown, op. cit., p. 193.
13. Howard Berliner, 'Scientific Medicine since Flexner', in JW Salmon (ed), *Alternative Medicines: Popular and policy perspectives*, p. 35.
14. For an account of the less savoury activities of IG Farben under Hitler's regime during the 1940s, see Josiah Dubois, *The Devil's Chemists*.
15. R Hare, *The Birth of Penicillin and the Disarming of Microbes*, p. 147.
16. Anselm Strauss and Juliet Corbin, *Shaping a New Health Care System*; see also Max Gerson, *A Cancer Therapy: Results of fifty cases*, pp. 167–85.
17. The Harvard Working Group on New and Resurgent Diseases, 'New and Resurgent Diseases: The failure of attempted eradication', *The Ecologist*, vol. 25, no. 1, January/February 1995, 21–26, p. 26.
18. Rene Dubos, *Mirage of Health: Utopias, progress and biological change*, p. 104.
19. Rene Dubos, in David Sobel, op. cit., pp. xii–xiii.
20. Ibid., pp. ix–x.
21. Maurice Pappworth, *Human Guinea Pigs: Experimentation on man*, pp. 221–2.
22. Ibid., p. 278.
23. J Harkness, S Lederer and D Wikler, 'Laying ethical foundations for clinical research', *Bulletin of the World Health Organization*, 2001, 79(4), 365–72, p. 365.
24. H Beecher, 'Ethics and Clinical Research', *The New England Journal of Medicine*, 1966, 274, 24, 1354–60, p. 1355. (Article reproduced in full in J Harkness et al, op. cit.)
25. Rick Carlson, *The End of Medicine*, pp. 210–11.
26. Ivan Illich, *Limits to Medicine: Medical nemesis. The expropriation of health*, pp. 135–6.
27. Richard Taylor, *Medicine Out of Control: The anatomy of a malignant technology*, p. 196.
28. Ibid., p. 237.

29. John Ehrenreich (ed), *The Cultural Crisis of Modern Medicine*, pp. 22–3.
30. Rick Carlson, op. cit., pp. 71–2.
31. Mike Saks, op. cit., p. 117.
32. Ian Gawler, *You Can Conquer Cancer*.
33. Michael Baum, 'Rationalism versus Irrationalism in the Care of the Sick: Science Versus the Absurd', *Medical Journal of Australia*, 1989, vol. 151, p. 607.
34. Edmund Pellegrino, 'The Sociocultural Impact of Twentieth Century Therapeutics', in Morris D Vogel and Charles E Rosenberg, *The Therapeutic Revolution*, p. 262.
35. Ibid., p. 264.
36. Larry Dossey, *Space, Time and Medicine*.
37. Larry Dossey, *Healing Words: The power of prayer and the practice of medicine*.
38. Kenneth Pelletier, *Sound Mind, Sound Body: A new model for lifelong health*.
39. Quoted in Franz Hartmann, *Paracelsus: Life and Prophecies*, p. 110.

Chapter 4

1. Rene Dubos, 'Preface' in David Sobel, *Ways of Health: Holistic approaches to ancient and contemporary medicine*, p. x.
2. Max Gerson, *A Cancer Therapy: Results of fifty cases*, p. 13.
3. Thomas McKeown, *The Role of Medicine: Dream, mirage, or nemesis?*, p. 6.
4. Helen Graham, *Time, Energy and the Psychology of Healing*, p. 28.
5. Andrew Taylor Still, *Autobiography*.
6. Rick Carlson, *The End of Medicine*, p. 210.
7. Marc Renaud, 'On the Structural Constraints to State Intervention in Health', in John Ehrenreich (ed), *The Cultural Crisis of Modern Medicine*, p. 108.
8. Thomas Kuhn, *The Structure of Scientific Revolutions*, p. 167.
9. Rachel Naomi Remen, *Kitchen Table Wisdom: Stories that heal*, p. 62.
10. Miriam Wetzel, Ted Kaptchuk, Aviad Haramati and David Eisenberg, 'Complementary and Alternative Medical Therapies: Implications for medical education', *Annals of Internal Medicine*, 2003, vol. 138, 3, 191–6; Victoria Maizes, Craig Schneider, Iris Bell and Andrew Weil, 'Integrative Medical Education: Development and Implementation of a Comprehensive Curriculum at the University of Arizona', *Academic Medicine*, 2002, vol. 77, 9, 851–60; Peter Brooks, 'Undergraduate Teaching of Complementary Medicine', *Medical Journal of Australia*, 2004, vol. 181 (5), p. 275.
11. Rick Carlson, *The End of Medicine*, p. 150; Ivan Illich, *Limits to Medicine: Medical nemesis. The expropriation of health*, pp. 255–6.
12. Helen Graham, op. cit., pp. 67–8.
13. Fritjof Capra, *The Turning Point: Science, society and the rising culture*, pp. 335–6.

14. Sudhir Kakar, *Shamans, Mystics and Doctors: A psychological inquiry into India and its healing traditions*, p. 31.

Chapter 5

1. Rosemary Taylor, 'Alternative Medicine and the Medical Encounter in Britain and the United States', in JW Salmon (ed), *Alternative Medicines: Popular and policy perspectives*, p. 205.
2. Eric Cassell, *The Healer's Art*, p. 114.
3. Ibid., p. 56.
4. Edmund Pellegrino, 'Towards an Expanded Medical Ethics: The Hippocratic Ethic Revisited', in Robert Veach (ed), *Cross Cultural Perspectives in Medical Ethics: Readings*, p. 32.
5. Michael Balint, *The Doctor, His Patient and the Illness*, p. 39.
6. Eric Cassell, op. cit., p. 48.
7. Thomas Szasz, *The Myth of Mental Illness*.
8. Carl Jung, *The Undiscovered Self; see also his *Memories, Dreams and Reflections*.
9. *See* RD Laing, *The Divided Self, Self and Others* and RD Laing and Aaron Esterton, *Sanity, Madness and the Family*. An informative overview of Laing and his group's activities with both supportive and critical commentaries is available through Robert Boyers and Robert Orrill's edited anthology *Laing and Anti-Psychiatry*.
10. Thomas Szasz and Marc Hollander, 'A Contribution to the Philosophy of Medicine: The basic models of the doctor–patient relationship', *AMA Archives of Internal Medicine*, 1956, vol. 97, pp. 585–92.
11. Ibid., p. 586.
12. Ibid., p. 587.
13. Eric Cassell, op. cit., p. 141.
14. Howard Stein, *The Psychodynamics of Medical Practice: Unconscious factors in patient care*, p. 58.
15. Thomas Szasz and Marc Hollander, op. cit., p. 588.
16. Ian McWhinney, *Being a General Practitioner: What it means*, p. 315.
17. Michael Balint, op. cit., p. 121.
18. Eric Cassell, op. cit., pp. 137–38.
19. Ibid., p. 74.
20. Rollo May, *The Art of Counselling*, p. 63.
21. Michael Balint, op. cit., pp. 107–8.
22. Eric Cassell, op. cit., p. 67.
23. Ibid., p. x.

Chapter 6

1. Thomas McKeown, *The Role of Medicine: Dream, mirage, or nemesis?*, p. xiv.
2. Fritjof Capra, *The Turning Point: Science, society and the rising culture*, p. 365.
3. Richard Taylor, *Medicine Out of Control: The anatomy of a malignant technology*, p. 39.
4. Quoted in Henry Sigerist (ed), *Four Treatises of Theophrastus von Hohenheim, Called Paracelsus*, p. 38.
5. Donald Moss, 'Psychotherapy and Human Experience', in Ronald Valle and Steen Halling, *Existential-Phenomenological Perspectives in Psychology: Exploring the breadth of human experience*, pp. 194–5.
6. Fritjof Capra, op. cit., p. 361.
7. Meredith McGuire, *Ritual Healing in Suburban America*, p. 235.
8. Helen Graham, *Time, Energy and the Psychology of Healing*, p. 19.
9. Jeanne Achterberg, 'The Shaman: Master Healer in the Imaginary Realm', in Shirley Nicholson (ed), *Shamanism: An expanded view of reality*, pp. 103–24.
10. Rene Dubos, *Mirage of Health: Utopias, progress and biological change*, p. 118.
11. Ivan Illich, *Limits to Medicine: Medical nemesis: The expropriation of health*, p. 61.
12. Paul Ghalioungui, *Magic and Medical Science in Ancient Egypt*, pp. 149–53.
13. Edmund Bordeaux Szekely, *The Essene Gospel of Peace: Book 1*.
14. Bernard Jensen, *Tissue Cleansing through Bowel Management*; Max Gerson, *A Cancer Therapy: Results of fifty cases*.
15. VB Dash, *Fundamentals of Ayurvedic Medicine*.
16. Vincent Di Stefano, 'Towards Regeneration', *Australian Journal of Medical Herbalism*, vol. 2, 3, 1990, pp. 55–8.
17. Wolfe Segal, 'Naturopathy, Homeopathy and Herbalism', in Richard Joske and Wolfe Segal, *Ways of Healing*, pp. 83–115.
18. Richard Taylor, op. cit., p. 22.
19. Kenneth Pelletier, *Sound Mind, Sound Body: A new model for lifelong health*, p. 25.
20. Meredith McGuire, op. cit., pp. 32–3.

Chapter 7

1. Jean Gebser, *The Ever-Present Origin*, p. 542.
2. Georg Feuerstein, *Structures of Consciousness: The genius of Jean Gebser. An introduction and critique*, p. 119.
3. See Peter Chojnowski, 'Descartes' Dream: From method to madness', *The Angelus*, XXV, no. 4, April 2002.
4. Lex Newman, 'Descartes' Epistemology', Section 7: 'Proving the existence of the external, material world'.

5. Betty Dobbs, *The Foundations of Newton's Alchemy: or, 'The Hunting of the Greene Lyon'*, p. 6.
6. Fielding H Garrison, *An Introduction to the History of Medicine*, p. 21.
7. Larry Dossey, *Time, Space and Medicine*, pp. 3–6.
8. Fritjof Capra, *The Turning Point: Science, society and the rising culture*, p. 350.
9. Lawrence Foss, 'A Challenge to Biomedicine: A foundations perspective', *Journal of Medicine and Philosophy*, vol. 14, pp. 168–9.
10. Ibid., p. 171.
11. Egon Guba, *The Paradigm Dialogue*, p. 17.
12. Carl Matheson, 'Historicist Theories of Rationality'.
13. Thomas Kuhn, *The Structure of Scientific Revolutions*, p. 84.
14. Arthur Kornberg, 'The Two Cultures: Chemistry and Biology', *Biochemistry*, 1987, vol. 26, pp. 6888–91. This article is adapted from Kornberg's Plenary Address to the American Association for the Advancement of Science given in February 1987.
15. EF Schumacher, *Small is Beautiful: A study of economics as if people mattered*, p. 85.
16. Psychiatrist Shafica Karagulla offers an in-depth portrayal of the perceptual world of Dora Kunz, to whom she gives the pseudonym Diane, in her study of various forms of clairvoyant perception *Breakthrough to Creativity*. See particularly pp. 124–61); *see also* Dolores Krieger, *The Therapeutic Touch: How to use your hands to help and heal*.
17. Terence and Dennis McKenna, *The Invisible Landscape*, p. 95.
18. Jan Smuts, *Holism and Evolution*, p. 176.
19. Shafica Karagulla, *Breakthrough to Creativity*, p. 78.
20. Meredith McGuire, *Ritual Healing in Suburban America*, p. 198.
21. Kendall Johnson, *The Living Aura: Radiation field photography and the Kirlian effect*, pp. 106–19.
22. Earle Lane, *Electrophotography*, p. 43.
23. HS Dakin, *High Voltage Photography*, pp. 26–33. Regarding the phenomenon of metal-bending, see the detailed and provocative study by UK experimental physicist John Hasted, *The Metal Benders*.
24. Rupert Sheldrake, *The Presence of the Past: Morphic resonance and the habits of nature*.
25. Thomas Kuhn, op. cit., p. 6.
26. Jean Gebser, *The Ever-Present Origin*, p. 542.
27. Jolande Jacobi, *Paracelsus: Selected writings*, pp. 63–4.

Chapter 8

1. Thomas Merton, *Conjectures of a Guilty Bystander*, p. 6.
2. Kenneth Pelletier, *Sound Mind, Sound Body: A new model for lifelong health*, p. 231.

3. Margaret Stacey, *The Sociology of Health and Healing*, p. 175.
4. Edmund Pellegrino, 'The Sociocultural Impact of Twentieth-Century Therapeutics', in Morris D Vogel and Charles E Rosenberg, *The Therapeutic Revolution*, p. 256.
5. Manfred Porkert, 'Chinese Medicine: A traditional healing science', in David Sobel, *Ways of Health: Holistic approaches to ancient and contemporary medicine*, p. 166.
6. Daniel Mowrey has documented many studies of traditional herbal medicines that have successfully passed through the hoops of formal scientific validation of efficacy. See his *The Scientific Validation of Herbal Medicine* and *Next Generation Herbal Medicine*.
7. Richard Smith, 'Foregone Conclusions: The public is being regularly deceived by the drug trials funded by pharmaceutical companies, loaded to generate the results they need', *The Guardian*, 14 January 2004.
8. Quoted by Carlo Calabrese, 'Clinical Research in Naturopathic Medicine', in George Lewith, Wayne Jonas and Harald Walach, *Clinical Research in Complementary Therapies: Principles, problems and solutions*, p. 358.
9. *British Herbal Pharmacopeia*; M Blumenthal, WR Busse, A Goldberg, et al (eds), *The Complete Commission E Monographs: Therapeutic guide to herbal medicines*.
10. A number of these assumptions are challenged by Harald Wallach, Wayne Jonas and George Lewith in their excellent review, 'The Role of Outcomes Research in Evaluating Complementary Medicine', *Alternative Therapies*, 2002, 8, 3, pp. 88–95. The article itself is reprinted from their anthology *Clinical Research in Complementary Therapies*, Churchill Livingstone, London 2001.
11. Meredith McGuire, *Ritual Healing in Suburban America*, p. 14.
12. Ibid., p. 13.
13. Ibid., p. 201.
14. Pelletier, op. cit., p. 26.
15. Ibid., p. 170.
16. Bruce Barrett and Lucille Marchand et al, 'What Complementary and Alternative Medicine Practitioners Say About Health and Health Care', *Ann. Fam. Med.*, 2004, vol. 2, pp. 253–9.
17. See Victoria Maizes, Craig Schneider, Iris Bell and Andrew Weil, 'Integrative Medical Education: Development and implementation of a comprehensive curriculum at the University of Arizona', *Academic Medicine*, 2002, vol. 77, 9, 851–60.
18. Iris Bell and Opher Caspi et al, 'Integrative Medicine and Systemic Outcomes Research: Issues in the emergence of a new model for primary health care', *Arch. Int. Med.*, 2002, vol. 162(2), pp. 133–40.
19. *See* Harold Wallach, Wayne Jonas and George Lewith, op. cit.
20. Thomas Kuhn, *The Structure of Scientific Revolutions*, p. 48.

21. Miriam Wetzel, Ted Kaptchuk, Aviad Haramati and David Eisenberg, 'Complementary and Alternative Medical Therapies: Implications for medical education', *Annals of Internal Medicine*, 2003, vol. 138, 3, pp. 191–6; Brian Berman, 'Complementary Medicine and Medical Education: Teaching complementary medicine offers a way of making teaching more holistic', *BMJ*, 2001, 322, pp. 121–2.

22. Ted Kaptchuk, 'The Placebo Effect in Alternative Medicine: Can the performance of a healing ritual have clinical significance?', *Annals of Internal Medicine*, 2002, vol. 136, pp. 817–25. *See also* the brilliant and humane reflections of medical homoeopath David Reilly's 'Some Reflections on Creating Therapeutic Consultations', in David Peters (ed) 2001, *Understanding the Placebo Effect in Complementary Medicine*, pp. 89–110.

Chapter 9

1. Rachel Naomi Remen, *Kitchen Table Wisdom*, p. 164.
2. Thomas Berry, *The Ecozoic Era*, p. 6.
3. K Alster, *The Holistic Health Movement*, pp. 172–3.
4. Paul Ghalioungui, *Magic and Medical Science in Ancient Egypt*, p. 153.
5. Vincent Di Stefano, 'Towards Regeneration', *Australian Journal of Medical Herbalism*, 1990, vol. 2, 3, pp. 55–8.
6. Steven Fulder, *The Handbook of Complementary Medicine*, p. 39.
7. Catherine Zollman and Andrew Vickers, 'ABC of Complementary Medicine: What is complementary medicine?', *BMJ*, 1999, vol. 319, pp. 693–6; 'Alternative Medicine' (theme issue), *JAMA*, 1998, vol. 280 (18), pp. 1549–640; 'Alternative Medicine' (section), *Med. J. Aust.*, 1998, vol. 169, pp. 573–86.
8. Bruce Wilcox, A Aguirre et al, 'EcoHealth: A transdisciplinary imperative for a sustainable future' (editorial), *EcoHealth*, 2004, vol. 1, pp. 3–5. *See also* Tony McMichael, 'The Biosphere, Health, and Sustainability' (editorial), *Science*, 2002, vol. 297, 16 August, p. 1093.
9. Thanks to the late Greg Ah Ket for alerting me to this story.
10. Thomas Berry, op. cit., p. 3.
11. Union of Concerned Scientists, *World Scientists' Warning to Humanity*.
12. Thomas Berry, *The University: Its response to the ecological crisis*.
13. See EF Schumacher, *Small Is Beautiful: A study of economics as if people mattered*; Barbara Ward and Rene Dubos, *Only One Earth: The care and maintenance of a small planet*; Rosalie Bertell, *No Immediate Danger: Prognosis for a radioactive earth*.
14. K Alster, op. cit., p. 44.

15. Mike Saks, *Orthodox and Alternative Medicine: Politics, professionalisation, and health care*, p. 108.

16. Rene Dubos, 'Hippocrates in Modern Dress', in David Sobel (ed), *Ways of Health: Holistic approaches to ancient and contemporary medicine*, pp. 205–20.

Index